A Collection of Essays from the Human Food Project

rewild

YOU'RE 99% MICROBE.
IT'S TIME YOU STARTED EATING LIKE IT.

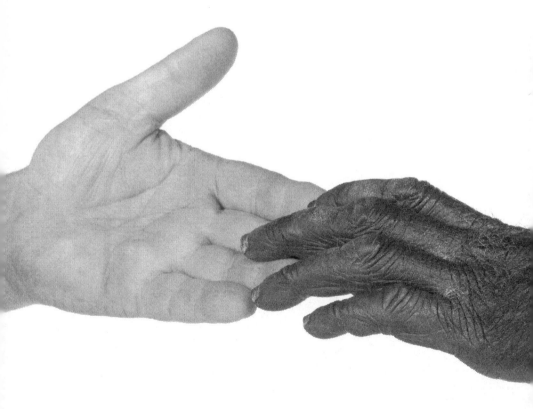

Jeff D. Leach

AUTHORS NOTE

This book is a collection of essays from the Human Food Project's website (www.humanfoodproject.com). That said, this is not a traditional book with an obvious beginning and end - but rather a collection of essays that share a common thread: the human microbiome.

100% of the proceeds from this book go to support our research in Africa and Mongolia.

OTHER TITLES BY THE AUTHOR

Honor Thy Symbionts

Bloom (forthcoming, Victory Belt Publishing)

Hadza: Field Notes from the Human Food Project (forthcoming, Human Food Project)

Also check out **humanfoodbar.com**

CONTENTS

rewild

A Fecal Transplant from a Healthy Chimpanzee or Average Joe – which would you choose?

PLAY ALONG FOR A MOMENT.

The year is 2020 and all hell has broken loose. You're part of a small band of people wandering the post-apocalyptic streets of downtown Atlanta, staying one step ahead of the flesh-eating 'walkers.' If spending all day trying to avoid being infected (or possibly eaten) by a zombie wasn't bad enough, months on the run drinking iffy water and eating what you could scrounge has taken its toll on your gut - or at least that's what you think. Most of the time you are doubled-over and good day is measured by your ability to keep the tiniest nibble of food in your gut. You're wasting away.

As luck would have it, your small band finds itself standing outside an unassuming building among a sea of unassuming buildings, slung across a sprawling campus on the outskirts of Atlanta. Ground zero - you have found The Center for Disease Control and its Primate Biomedical Research Center - aka 'chimp asylum.' After some discussion, sympathetic researchers inside grant you entrance.

If government employees who specialize in the world's nastiest infectious diseases know how to do anything, it's how to hunker down during a zombie apocalypse. Completely self-contained with their own water supply, electricity and a pile of shelf stable food, the group of a dozen researchers could probably make it a few years if need be, or however long it takes Will Smith and Bruce Willis to solve a little zombie problem.

Amid the various offices and laboratories in the building are rows of caged chimpanzees 'participating' in biomedical research. Throughout the zombie ordeal, the researchers have dutifully cared for the animals, continuing daily feeding and medications. Amazingly, in the center of the building sits a lush, park-like enclosure half the size of a football field. Amongst the trees and dense tropical-like foliage, (maintained with mechanically controlled humidity and rainfall), are two-dozen common chimpanzees (*Pan troglodytes*) roaming about eating foods that are familiar. This recent population had been captured near Gombe in Tanzania. They had arrived at the CDC days before the zombie invasion and had not transitioned into the biomedical program - yet.

One of your new hosts notices that you are ill and queries your problem, (it seems your two visits to the bathroom in an hour gave you away). After listening to you recount your symptoms, one of the researchers who had gathered with the others to hear your story suggests you might have a nasty bug, possibly even *Clostridium difficile* - or C Diff as it is otherwise known. He asks if you had been hospitalized recently or taken broad-spectrum antibiotics, either of which (or a combination of) could be contributing to your problem. Turns out days before the apocalypse you had some minor surgery at a local hospital and had taken not only one course of antibiotics, but several.

As the days wore on at chimp asylum, your frequent visits to the bathroom had only gotten worse, even after the researchers had given you more antibiotics. The antibiotics in fact, had only made things much worse. One of the researchers - a microbiologist tasked with screening stool samples from new chimps for problematic viruses and pathogens using metagenomic tools - suggests that you might consider a 'fecal transplant.'

As the name implies, a 'fecal transplant' is just that. Following a high-volume enema deep into your colon (from the business end of your GI tract) to clean things out, a small sample of a donor stool from a (presumably) healthy individual is inserted. (Nasogastric tube from the top end is used in some instances - more of a European thing). The donor sample teeming with trillions of (presumably) healthy bacterial cells then sets up shop in your colon. Balance is then reinstated in an ecosystem sent into a tailspin by the opportunistic pathogen(s) that bloomed following a perturbation - presumably from the scorched earth effect of said broad-spectrum antibiotics. By doing a number on the diversity and abundance of microbes in your gut - both friend and foe and everything in between - broad-spectrum antibiotics have the potential to significantly shift the composition[1] of your gut microbial community and provide opportunities for low abundance pathogens to rise up. As mounting research[2] suggests, fecal transplants are impressively effective in solving recurrent C. diff infections - one such opportunistic pathogen.

Given your current state and the researcher's explanation of the procedure (along with his assurance he could pull it off), as well as the evidence to support its potential success in solving your problem, the only question remaining is who the donor would be? More to the point, how do you define a healthy gut microbiome in a potential donor, especially among a rag tag bunch of apocalyptic survivors just trying to make it to the next day? Do you pick the older guy, the 20-something female you been traveling with or maybe her 14-year old little brother? The Mexican guy looks healthy, but so does the Asian couple - though he's a bit on the heavy side. But does that even matter? What about the researchers? A mixed bag of gender, age, body-type, race and attitude - could one of them would be suitable?

Maybe you could ask the potential donors for a sample of test poo for the microbiologist to evaluate - you're in a biomedical research facility after all. The pre-screening of samples with high-throughput sequencing technology would provide a snapshot of the microbes in the guts of your comrades and allow you to weed out any obvious bad donors based on the nasty bugs they may be carrying. Yet alas, while the researcher has all the equipment to pull this off, they had run out of some critical supplies just before the coming of the 'walkers' and had not been resupplied. Pre-screening was out.

As you scan over the faces and bellies of your potential donors the doe-eyed primate handler blurts out, *"What about one of the chimps that just came in from Tanzania?"* A little taken back at first, you press your face to the glass of the football field sized jungle enclosure and consider the possibility.

Even though we differ in some aspects of appearance and behavior, humans share 99% of the same DNA[3] with

4

common chimpanzees (and about the same with their close cousins the bonobo as it turns out). When you consider that some of those DNA differences are responsible for things like hair and sensory perception[4] and have nothing to do with diet and immunity (and microbes), we are even more similar than the 99% figure suggests.

Short of the tranquilizer shot into their rump back in Tanzania, the chimps in the jungle enclosure had not been exposed to any medication or funky monkey chow fed to the chimps already enrolled in the biomedical program. To ease the transition into Western life and biomedical research, they were enjoying (as much as a captive chimp could) their familiar foods and vegetation within the enclosure. These chimps were as close to pure or untainted as any chimp could be in Atlanta - or anywhere in the US for that matter - and lucky for you, the first thing the microbiologist did when the new batch of chimps arrived was to collect stool samples and analyze them. No nasty viruses and nothing out of the ordinary just pure, unadulterated monkey poo from the birthplace of humanity; East Africa.

You weigh up the pros and cons. As with humans, 80-90% of all the bacteria in the chimp gut belong to[5] the major phyla of *Firmicutes* and *Bacteroidetes*. As with chimps, humans have simple guts and like other mammalian fermenters, our gut microbes are necessary to break down and release sugars from plant polysaccharides. We are also omnivores - in that we eat plants and animals. So too are chimps. In fact, the chimps currently in jungle asylum are from the Gombe region of Tanzania, made famous by Jane Goodall. Like all chimps, the Gombe chimps hunt and kill other animals including bushpig, bushbuck, rodents, birds, baboons and even other chimpanzees (plus the occasional human infant), but at the top of the menu

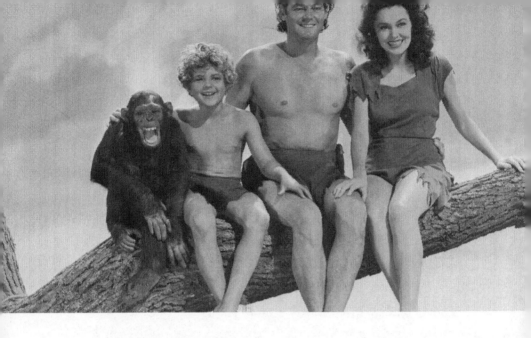

are the abundant red colobus monkeys. Though the amount of hunting and meat consumption among chimp communities throughout Africa varies, based on habitat and access to prey (and from season to season), it can reach staggering levels. During one season in 1992, the chimp community at Gombe[6] (45 individuals) successfully killed more than 1,300 pounds of red colobus, bushpigs and bushbucks, (which included more than 100 red colobus monkeys). Given the researchers are unable to witness every hunt, the estimates for 1992 are thought to be much higher.

As pointed out[7] by anthropologist and primate researcher Craig Stanford, *"The percentage of the chimpanzee diet that is meat is therefore quite substantial and approaches the figures for the low end of the range of some human foragers."* On top of that, in the west-African country of Senegal, savannah chimps are known to fashion sticks into spears[8] to hunt and kill small, nocturnal bushbabies. Good heavens, a Charlton Heston-like nightmare come true!

Even below the phylum level, we share many of the

same genus level bacteria with chimps including *Bacteroides, Prevotella, Faeocalbacterium, Dialester, Bifidobacterium, Ruminococcus* and so on. Though there are differences in human-chimp immunity[9] associated with susceptibility to infectious diseases, chimps and humans share the same adaptive immunity, which tolerates the presence of select gut microbial communities and is rooted deep in our shared evolutionary past.

The variability in the gut microbes of humans is tremendous, people from Malawi[10] don't look much like people from the U.S., kid's guts in Burkina Faso[11] look different to kids from Italy, and while you might share 99.9% of the DNA with your neighbor down the street, your gut microbiomes can be as much as 80-90% unique. In other words, as the Human Microbiome Project and other such projects teach us that genetics can contribute to the shaping the composition of your gut microbiota, environmental factors such as diet and lifestyle play a fundamentally significant role. That said, while there are differences in the gut microbiota of chimps and humans - geography, diet and lifestyle may be contributing to those differences - more so than the underlying genetics which we more or less share anyway.

So, who shall your poo donor be? Among the human choices, you have to give serious thought to the inescapable fact that every single person standing before you was born and raised in a world of medications, chlorinated water, antibiotics, chemicals and funky, weird diets unknown to our ancestors and their microbes. As Westerners, we spend 90% of our time inside our homes, offices and cars, walled off from the natural world and its diverse metacommunity of microbes. By reducing our exposure to the *terra firma* of nature and its microbes and carpet-bombing our guts with medications and monotonous diets (by evolutionary standards), we likely harbor a less diverse and thus less *resilient* gut microbiome of any generation in human history. All of us - every last one of us - are in varying stages of gut dysbiosis. In fact, we may be so compromised as a generation that any attempt to model a normal or optimal gut microbiome from our ranks might be seen as a kind of 'fool's errand.'

Back to our future predicament. Months hunkering down (or on the run) from the zombie hoards appears to be taking its toll on the group as a whole, further calling into question the appropriateness of any of these humans as a potential donor. Your choice might (and should) start becoming easier. I also put this question of *healthy chimp versus sick human* to Jonathan Eisen[12], a microbiologist who works on the ecology and evolution of microbial communities at UC-Davis, though in our e-mail exchange we didn't define what 'sick' was in a human or how one defines 'healthy' in a chimp, nevertheless his conclusion was:

"Given the incredibly close relationship we have with chimps, I think it is reasonable to hypothesize that a healthy person might have more similarities in the microbiome with a healthy chimp than with a sick person. Therefore, I would choose to get my FT [Fecal Transplant] if I needed it from a chimp rather than from a sick person."

So next time you are at the zoo (maybe one that houses chimps just off the boat from Africa that have not been westernized in anyway - probably not at all likely), and you find yourself on the receiving end of some poo flying your way - you might like to catch a handful, take it home and pop it the freezer because you just never know when the zombie apocalypse might hit.

From Meat to Microbes to Main Street: is it time to trade in your George Foreman Grill?

IF SCIENTISTS KEEP PUBLISHING THE RESULTS of their work in journals human beings will be in danger of running out of stuff to eat. The latest nutritional 'no-no' literally has meat-eaters on the ropes, following a startling article published in *Nature Medicine*[13] that draws a *possible* link between the nutrient carnitine[14] (found in red meat) and cardiovascular disease. But what makes this interesting, (and so different from past debates - like how saturated fat and meat was once thought[15] to hasten your arrival at the pearly gates), is the role of gut microbes as an intermediary in this tangled web of cardiac arrest.

The story goes something like this: your run-of-the-mill 8-ounce steak contains ~180mg of the nutrient carnitine. In and of itself, carnitine is not a bad thing. Your body produces it naturally and it's used everyday in the transport of fatty acids into your mitochondria. *Dietary carnitine*, however, comes from a slab of red meat that can be gobbled up (metabolized) by your resident gut bacteria and converted into something called TMA (trimethylamine). So far so good, until it diffuses and makes its way from your gut into the serum (blood). Since TMA is a gas at room (and body) temperature, translocating across the gut barrier is not a problem. Once in your blood, TMA makes its way to your liver where it's oxidized into TMAO (trimethylamine-*N*-oxide). From this point, the researchers argue that elevated levels of TMAO muddy up some mechanisms including cholesterol transport, which then accelerates atherosclerosis. In short, not good news for red meat lovers, or so it might seem.

This is a complicated paper with a lot of moving parts that are worth (re)considering, yet the most interesting finding is the role of gut bacteria in this process. The data presented in the paper suggests that vegans and vegetarians have a decreased capacity to generate TMA from dietary carnitine than do omnivores, due to the simple fact they harbor different gut bacteria. The most striking finding in this bacterial connection and the one that almost caused me to fall out of my chair, was the role of one group of bacteria known as *Prevotella*. The researchers discovered that regardless of whether you were a vegan/vegetarian or an omnivore, higher levels of *Prevotella* in your gut correlated with higher levels of TMAO in your blood. Using gut microbial data from three individuals recently analyzed as part of the American Gut[16] project - one of which is myself - I will touch upon the irony of the argument that 'carnivorous habits' may lead to accelerated atherosclerosis in the context of *Prevotella*. But first, lets look at the *Nature Medicine* paper.

To demonstrate that gut bacteria are necessary to

convert carnitine from red meat to TMA in the gut, which if you remember is then absorbed into the blood, making its way to the liver where it is further converted into TMAO, researchers gathered together five omnivores and fed them each an 8-ounce sirloin steak (which contains ~180mg of carnitine) and a tablet of an additional 250mg of carnitine (d3-carnitine), tagged with a heavy isotope which allowed the researchers to follow this particular dose through the body. So we have regular (dietary) carnitine from the red meat and an isotope labeled d3-carnitine (note the d3 denotes isotope labeled). The researchers then drew blood after the meal over a period of 24 hours and as expected, the levels of d3-TMAO went up over time, indicating that the gut bacteria did their thing and metabolized the isotopic d3-carnitine into d3-TMA that was absorbed and converted to d3-TMAO by the liver. Interestingly, while the d3-carnitine from the tablet ended up as d3-TMAO in serum, the native (or natural) carnitine and TMAO from the steak only showed 'modest' concentrations in the serum, according to the researchers. In other words, the impact of the steak was semi-uneventful.

To further demonstrate the contribution of gut bacteria to the carnitine>TMA>TMAO development, the researchers put the same five omnivores who wolfed down the sirloin steak with the 250mg carnitine chaser on broad-spectrum antibiotics for a week (metronidazole 500mg and ciprofloxacin 500mg – twice daily) to suppress their gut bacteria, as broad-spectrum antibiotics have a tendency to do[17]. After taking antibiotics twice a day for a week, the 5 omnivores were called back in and given another 8-ounce sirloin steak and 250mg d3-carnitine tablet. However, unlike during the first visit, the week of antibiotics caused a 'near complete suppression' of TMAO in blood or urine. On top of that, no d3-TMAO was noted either.

In other words, no detectable levels of TMAO or d3-TMAO were formed, suggesting that whatever bacteria were present before that were endowed with the genes to metabolize carnitine from meat or the tablet into TMA, were gone.

After this second meal at the end of the week of antibiotics, the researchers discontinued the antibiotics and sent the omnivore's home. After a few weeks had passed (and enough time had presumably lapsed for their gut microbiota to recover from the 'week of antibiotic hell'), the omnivores were called back in for another steak and 250mg tablet. This time, the gut bacteria that were capable of metabolizing carnitine into TMA in the gut had reappeared as TMAO and d3-TMAO came back with a vengeance in the blood and urine. Taken together, all three steak dinners and tablet chasers demonstrate that the 'TMAO production from dietary carnitine in humans is dependent on intestinal microbiota.'

At this point you're probably wondering which bacteria were depleted during the week of antibiotics and who were the nasty culprits responsible for creating TMA (but were metabolically shut down during a week of broad-spectrum antibiotics only to re-bloom after the fog of antibiotic war had lifted?). It would seem simple enough to say that they were there during the first meal, wiped out during the week of antibiotics and then reappeared after several weeks of recovery. As amazing as it might sound, it appears the researchers DID NOT collect stool samples during this phase of the project and so have very little idea as to how the microbial composition had shifted before, during and after antibiotics. How unfortunate.

At this point the researchers noted that TMAO (native and d3-labeled) varied among individuals following the ingestion of carnitine. More to the point, a *post-hoc* nutritional

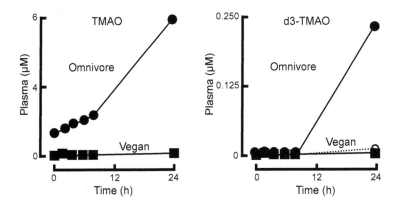

Figure adapted from: Koeth RA, Wang Z, Levison BS, et al. Intestinal microbiota metabolism of L-carnitine, a nutrient in red meat, promotes atherosclerosis. Nature Medicine. 2013;19(5):576-585.

survey revealed that red meat consumption might actually enhance one's ability to generate TMAO from carnitine, so it was time to break out the George Foreman Grill again, get some tablets of carnitine ready and invite a vegan round to dinner. (Kudos to the researchers for getting a long-term (>5 years) vegan to chow down an 8-ounce sirloin steak (plus the additional 250mg of d3-carnitine)).

The figure above plots what happened next. Over the course of 24 hours they took several blood samples from the vegan. As you can see, no appreciable amounts of TMAO showed up in the blood as a result of ingesting the steak (left panel) or the isotope-laden d3-TMAO for that matter (right panel). Keep in mind this is a sample size of exactly ONE person. For comparison, the researchers also plotted a 'single representative omnivore' who self-reported eating meat on a daily basis. Though the researchers did not specify, the assumption is that the data plotted below for this 'single representative omnivore' is from one of the five omnivores that participated in the previous five-omnivore study discussed above.

That said, among the five omnivores to choose from it's not exactly clear which omnivore they selected to plot against the vegan. Was it the one with the largest concentrations of TMAO, the one with the least amount or was it one from the middle of the pack? If it were me I would probably select the one with the greatest concentrations of TMAO to plot against the vegan, for dramatic effect. You see some of this 'dramatic effect' in the plot on the right (d3-TMAO). You will also notice that the panel on the left (TMAO) has vertical axis ticks set at 0, 4, and 6 - clearly showing a spike in the level of TMAO for the omnivore. However, the panel on the right (d3-TMAO) has the ticks on the vertical axis set at 0, 0.125 and 0.250 to create a pretty dramatic effect for one that really didn't exist. I have taken the liberty and re-plotted (dotted line) the concentrations of d3-TMAO for the omnivore the researchers had used the same vertical scale as the panel on left. This is much less dramatic and clearly shows that in a sample size of exactly ONE for each group (omnivore vs vegan), the omnivore showed elevated levels of native TMAO and a rather nominal increase of d3-TMAO from the isotope-laden pill. In other words, the gut microbiota from both individuals failed to metabolize the 250mg of d3-carnitine into meaningful levels of d3-TMAO in the blood.

As a side note, it's also not clear if the TMAO levels for the 'represented omnivore' are from baseline (pre-antibiotics) or the TMAO levels measured during the third visit - the one following the several weeks of washout to allow the gut microbiota of the five individuals to recover. I'm not being nit picky here, but this does matter (quite a lot). It matters as the researchers note in the Supplemental Data that a 'representative omnivore' has significantly greater levels of TMAO in their blood after the weeks of washout from the antibiotics over baseline - we don't know about the others. The assumption is that the gut microbiota of all five individuals had returned to its pre-antibiotic diversity and abundance, but we don't know for sure, as previous studies on the antibiotic impact of the gut microbiome have shown that it can take weeks (or even months) for the gut microbiome to recover and that it often settles back in a different composition altogether. All we know is that our five omnivores - based on one representative omnivore - had bounced back with a greater metabolic ability to yield TMA from dietary carnitine.

In either case it would be nice to know how 'representative' the omnivore actually was, and whether or not we are seeing the TMAO levels from a highly perturbed gut microbiota following antibiotic treatment. Increased gut permeability might be contributing to elevated TMAO levels as well. This, taken together with the sample size of ONE for each and the fact that no appreciable amount of d3-TMAO was noted among either (only TMAO for the omnivore), leaves me thinking that the jury is still out on this one. Fascinating nonetheless, but more data is needed. Sample of ONE does not allow for any statistical comparisons. Again unfortunate, but let's move on.

Here's where the study gets really interesting. This time the researchers gathered together 26 vegans & vegetarians and 51 omnivores (note in the text of the article the researchers say 23 vegans & vegetarians but show 26 in the plot below, so I will go with the 26). After fasting overnight for 12 hours, the researchers found that baseline levels of TMAO in the morning was significantly lower in the vegans & vegetarians compared to the omnivores (see figure left panel). However, there is

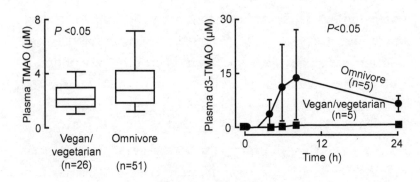

Figure adapted from: Koeth RA, Wang Z, Levison BS, et al. Intestinal microbiota metabolism of L-carnitine, a nutrient in red meat, promotes atherosclerosis. Nature Medicine. 2013;19(5):576-585.

considerable overlap in the box plots i.e. a considerable range. It appears there are vegans & vegetarians who had just as high (or higher) levels of TMAO than some omnivores. Given there are less vegans & vegetarians in the sample (26 vs 51), one wonders if increasing the sample of vegans & vegetarians to the same as the omnivores (n=51) would change this plot in anyway, possibly capturing more vegan/vegetarian variability?

From the 26 vegans & vegetarians and 51 omnivores the researchers picked five from each group and gave them each the 250mg d3-carnitine tablet (with no steak this time) and measured the d3-TMAO in the blood at several time points over 24 hours (see plot above). As can be seen, the d3-TMAO levels went up in the omnivores but not in the vegans & vegetarians. It's striking to see the variability in the omnivores, ranging from near zero to almost 30. Said differently, a SINGLE omnivore among the five can explain much of the elevated levels shown in the plot. Also, since this was a subset of the larger group of 26 vegans and vegetarians and 51 omnivores, we do not know if the researchers selected omnivores that showed higher levels of baseline (fasting) TMAO. Since they had to pick someone, it would be nice to know the selection criteria, i.e. did they pick omnivores with low, medium or higher levels of baseline TMAO levels? In either case, following the d3-carnitine challenge omnivores showed an increase as a group, but with some less so than others.

To explore the possibility that plasma TMAO levels might be associated with specific gut microbial taxa, the researchers collected stool samples from 23 of the 26 vegans & vegetarians and 30 of the 51 omnivores (at baseline). Sequencing the gene encoding for bacterial 16S rRNA of the stool samples, the researchers found some interesting patterns. As diet can significantly shape the composition of your gut microbiota - and differences between vegetarians have been noted in previous studies[18] - the resulting microbial differences were not completely unexpected. However, one particular group of bacteria did stand out; *Prevotella*. When the researchers grouped all 53 people (see plot next page) and analyzed them into so-called enterotypes (regardless of diet), they found that individuals that had gut microbiota enriched with *Prevotella* had higher levels of TMAO in their blood. Conversely, those with gut microbiota enriched with *Bacteroides* showed much lower levels of TMAO. While the concept of enterotypes is a matter of debate[19], *Prevotella*-enrichment remains evident for those levels of TMAO.

Interestingly, previous studies have suggested that enriched levels of *Prevotella* are associated with a higher carbohydrate diet, i.e. less meat. However, three of the four individuals (see plot) in the *Prevotella*-enriched group were meat eaters and the fourth was a vegan/vegetarian. On the flipside, of the 49 that clustered together - more *Bacteroides*, less *Prevotella* - was a mix of the omnivores and vegans & vegetarians. These

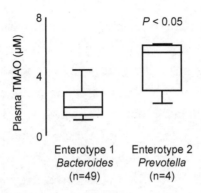

Figure adapted from: Koeth RA, Wang Z, Levison BS, et al. Intestinal microbiota metabolism of L-carnitine, a nutrient in red meat, promotes atherosclerosis. Nature Medicine. 2013;19(5):576-585.

findings suggest that previous dietary habits can drive microbial composition in the gut, which in turn affects the ability of your microbial ability to synthesize TMA/TMAO from dietary carnitine.

The potential role of *Prevotella* as a key player in this saga is made more interesting when you consider the results of feeding d3-carnitine to mice. In a series of experiments the researchers spiked the chow of a set of mice and compared the gut microbiota to a different group of mice receiving the same chow but without the d3-carnitine. You guessed it, the mice receiving the d3-carnitine had significantly higher levels of *Prevotella* as well as unclassified *Prevotellaceae*. Since the chow was the same between the two groups of mice, the carnitine seems to have the unique ability to nudge along the growth of *Prevotella* as well. More specifically, *Prevotella spp.* appear to harbor the genes necessary to synthesize carnitine, though the microbiota between mice and humans are not directly comparable, it is still interesting.

Quick side note: in an attempt to demonstrate that

carnitine is linked to heart disease, the researchers fed two groups of mice normal chow and spiked the water of one group with carnitine, which resulted in a doubling of atherosclerotic plaque and a 'doubling of disease burden' in the carnitine group at the end of 10 weeks. This part of the paper got a lot of attention from the popular press and was held up (along with other pieces in the *Nature Medicine* paper) as 'proof' that dietary carnitine from red meat can lead to accelerated atherosclerosis. However, what the article failed to mention was that the mice used in the study (*Apoe -/-* mice) are genetically engineered to be prone to atherosclerosis. On top of that, the 1.3% of carnitine in the drinking water is the equivalent to a human eating ~1,000 steaks a day[20]. You can decide for yourself if you think mice that are genetically engineered to be inclined to atherosclerosis who are fed the human equivalent of an entire cow every three days for 10 weeks is proof that carnitine from red meat accelerates atherosclerosis in humans.

The researchers also investigated the possible relationship of carnitine and cardiovascular disease in a cohort of 2,595 men and women undergoing *elective cardiac evaluation*. In short, they found an association between TMAO concentrations in serum and 'cardiovascular event risks.' They found the TMAO/cardiovascular risk the highest in the fourth quartile - or 650 of the 2,595 individuals. The average age of this group/quartile was 61 - 80% were male who were overweight to obese on average, one out of three had diabetes, 75% were hypertensive and a whopping 77% were smokers. Numerous medications like statins and beta-blockers were the norm and every biomarker of a crappy diet was elevated, as well as biomarkers of inflammation. In short, these folk were a mess.

It's important to note the TMAO association was just that - an association - and one among many. At this point it might be useful to mention that even though the researchers were focused on red meat, an amazing assortment of foods can generate levels of TMAO higher than that reported for red meat. To name a few: potatoes, peas, peanuts, eggs, mushrooms, bread, squid, prawn, crab, halibut, cod, herring, tuna and an assortment of other fishy things. So who's to say that red meat is responsible for the higher concentrations of TMAO in the sickest quartile of these 2,595 people? If a TMAO association is the issue then we might want to start issuing warnings to the general public that omega-rich fish are now off the menu, as well as carrots and peas. Remember, correlation does not equal causation.

The research in the *Nature Medicine* paper is important, as it clearly shows that gut bacteria are needed in the conversion of carnitine to TMA/TMAO. This was demonstrated when antibiotic-treated humans and mice were unable to produce TMAO after antibiotics were taken for a week but when they were discontinued the ability was restored and even enhanced. N.b. I did not discuss the antibiotic treatment in mice as it showed more or less what was seen in the human experiment. Unfortunately, the researchers did not collect stool samples so were unable to determine which bacteria were suppressed during the antibiotic treatment, but the role of bacteria in TMAO creation and TMAO as a risk factor or cause of atherosclerosis is a separate issue. If higher concentrations of TMAO (from unknown sources) are associated with an elevated risk of heart disease in a terribly sick group of predominantly adult males and mice genetically at risk for heart disease (fed the human equivalent of a cow every three days) is proof that TMAO causes atherosclerosis in the rest of us, then we might have a smoking gun, but I'm not so sure. I will leave that up to the statisticians and biochemistry propeller heads to sort out.

If we assume for the moment that TMAO can accelerate atherosclerosis, then the observation that enriched levels of *Prevotella* are associated with higher levels of TMAO become even more interesting, especially as enrichment of this group of bacteria seems to occur in vegans & vegetarians as well as omnivores. So what causes the enrichment of *Prevotella*? In a paper published in 2010, Italian researchers found that rural African kids in Burkina Faso had super high levels of *Prevotella*, while a similar aged group of kids in suburban Italy had none.

The striking dietary difference between the kids in Burkina Faso and the Italian kids was *whole grain consumption*. As with many rural African communities, grains - in this case millet and sorghum - are processed manually by stone grinding. Minus any winnowing process afterwards, these whole grains made up >50% of the daily calories in the village. In addition, they ate some legumes (black-eyed peas), some mango fruit, some butter and a very limited amount of vegetables. All in all, this is a very monotonous diet dominated by whole grains with very little diversity of anything else. In contrast, the Italian kids got ~25% of their daily calories from highly processed bread, biscuits, pasta and rice. The Italian kids also consumed legumes, a range of vegetables, milk, chicken, beef, fish, cod, sole, eggs, extra-virgin olive oil, butter, yogurt, cheese, snacks and a diversity of fruits - a much more diverse diet, though apparently devoid of any whole grains and high in processed foods.

As mentioned, the Italian kids had no traceable amounts of *Prevotella* in their stool samples. Below is a figure showing seven of the kids from Burkina Faso plotted below against two other individuals (Mr. A & B) & myself, recently sequenced as part of the American Gut project. While the sequencing data between American Gut and the African study are not directly comparable (different lab protocols etc), they are informative enough for this comparison.

While all of the kids from Burkina Faso showed very high levels of *Prevotella* (~>50%), the seven in the graph are the highest. In fact, the *Prevotella* levels among these Burkina Faso kids are among some of the highest reported for a cohort anywhere in the world. On left you see my *Prevotella* levels are 1.5%, Mr. A is at 0% and Mr. B at 32%. Interestingly, neither myself or Mr. A were eating much bread, pasta or any other grain-based foods. In my house, we get an artisan loaf of bread every few weeks to make sandwiches and occasionally eat bread when dining out, but I can't think of the last time I had pasta at home. Likewise, Mr. A avoids all processed foods, eats a lot

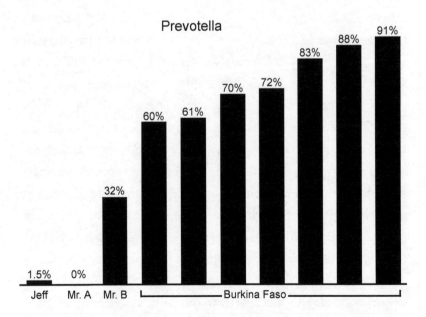

of fish and occasionally some beef. In short, he follows a Paleo diet. I too follow more or less a Paleo diet but not for ancestral reasons *per se*, my reasoning is more due to the fact that I have a type 1 diabetic daughter so I am hyper aware of the insulin spiking effects of processed foods.

As for Mr. B, an email exchange reveals a *very* diverse diet of plants and animals but a taste for whole wheat and whole grain foods in general, including whole oats for breakfast. Mr. B cooks often with whole wheat and whole grain ingredients. All three of us are of average BMI and physically active.

In the Burkina Faso paper, the researchers attributed the high levels of *Prevotella* to grain-based carbohydrates and most specifically; dietary fiber intake. While I personally do not eat grains on a regular basis, I do eat an extraordinary diversity of plants and thus have a high fiber intake - and yet low to no *Prevotella*. I would say some weeks I average 40-80g a day of dietary fiber from a range of foods. I go out of my way to try and consume a diversity of dietary fiber sources. Mr. A also eats lots of dietary fiber, but not from grain sources. That said, it doesn't appear that dietary fiber in general is driving the enrichment of the *Prevotella*. If it were, both myself and Mr. A would have higher levels of *Prevotella*. It appears somehow specific to the starch or dietary fiber in grains.

Prevotella, a gram-negative bacteria, are a common member of rumen and also present in high numbers in pigs, poultry and evidently, some humans. A recent genome analysis[21] of two common *Prevotella* (*P. ruminicola* and *P. bryantii*) reveals that they possess an extensive repertoire of genes targeted towards the degradation of non-cellulosic polysaccharides, such as hemicellulose and pectin - which is present in the cell walls of grasses and cereals (aka grains). While they can also utilize starches and simple sugars, they have also carved out a specific ecological niche when it comes to chomping down on the cell wall of grains. Think bran.

Interestingly, in a study[22] of 51 obese Finnish adults fed either a fiber-rich rye bread (whole grain) or a highly refined wheat bread for 12 weeks, those consuming the highly processed bread (no whole grain) showed a 37% decrease in the phylum Bacteroidetes, which includes genus *Prevotella*. Suggesting further that something particular to the whole grain - presumably the bran in the intact grain - is potentially modulating levels of *Prevotella*. However, another study[23] by the folks at the University of Nebraska didn't show much movement (up *or* down) in the abundance of *Prevotella* in 28 healthy individuals eating either whole-grain barley or brown rice. This same research group[24] also fed resistant starch (RS2 and RS4) in the form of crackers to ten people and saw nothing exciting with the abundance of *Prevotella*, suggesting (at least in this small study) that resistant starch (like that found in grains) does affect levels of *Prevotella*.

It's also worth noting that we see higher levels (15-30% of bacteria) of *Prevotella* among the San Bushmen in Namibia, who have shifted from hunting and gathering to more westernized foods, such as porridge made from goat's milk and whole-grain maize meal (as yet unpublished data from our work in Africa). Colleagues working among Amerindians in South America have noted elevated levels of *Prevotella* among more traditional groups eating lots of cassava. The contribution of other agricultural products is less clear, but overall it suggests some interesting patterns with this widely used root food.

I reached out to the researchers who published the *Nature Medicine* paper and asked if they might share the taxonomic summaries of the stool samples from the individuals in the study. They were kind enough to do so. Also known as an OTU table (Operational Taxonomic Units), the table breaks down the relative abundance of bacteria identified to the genus level. The OTU table revealed an abundance of *Prevotella* for the *Prevotella-enriched* group (enterotype discussed above) that included one vegan and three omnivores ranged from 16-54%. The highest abundance recorded (54%) was for the vegan. At 54%, that puts this particular individual in the same ballpark as the kids in Burkina Faso, and as for the rest, at least within the range of our whole grain-pasta-bread eating Mr. B.

So taken together, enriched levels of *Prevotella* appear to be associated with intake of whole-grain products but not necessarily associated with high fiber intake from non-grain plant sources, otherwise Paleo-like eaters like myself and Mr. A would have higher levels. Interestingly, the OTU table from the researchers revealed that the vast majority of vegans & vegetarians in the study had low to zero levels of *Prevotella*. I'm going to go out on a limb here and suggest that if vegans & vegetarians are anything, they are *starch eaters*. If starch that escapes digestion in the upper GI (resistant starch from amylose and amylopectin in grains) were driving *Prevotella* enrichment, then we would expect higher levels of *Prevotella* across this entire veggie cohort - but we didn't see this. This leaves the possible interpretation that the vegans & vegetarians who *didn't* show elevated levels of *Prevotella* are not heavy whole-grain eaters.

One last thing of interest with the kids from Burkina Faso: in addition to high levels of *Prevotella*, they also exhibited high levels of a genus known as *Xylanibacter* (which was absent in our biscuit and pasta eating Italian kids). As the '*Xylan*' in *Xylanibacter* implies, it's especially adept at degrading the xylan found in plant wall cells, similar to those found in whole grains. Below is the levels of *Prevotella* (bottom axis) plotted against

25

the levels of *Xylanibacter* in the subjects in the *Nature Medicine* paper along with some addition data from another study[25]. While the overall abundance of *Xylanibacter* is low compared to the African kids, the plant cell wall metabolizer *Xylanibacter* goes up as the abundance of *Prevotella* goes up. Taken together with the whole-grain-based diet of the Burkina Faso kids, the co-occurrence of these genera might have something to do with their whole-grain consumption.

To wrap it up, I'm not sure what to make of the carnitine-induced atherosclerosis in the heart attack prone mice fed the equivalent of mountains of red meat. I'm also not sure what to make of the sample size of ONE, that compared the newly meat-eating vegan to a 'representative omnivore.' Hopefully future studies will shed some light on this. It's also important to note the researchers never tested meat alone and that it was always red meat *and* d3-carnitine and whilst I'm not

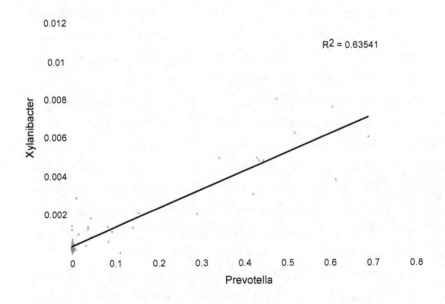

sure if it matters, it also might. I do like the clear demonstration that gut bacteria play a role in TMAO formation, as antibiotic treatment for a week shifted the gut microbiota just enough to blunt down the bacteria and the genes capable of metabolizing carnitine. It's just unfortunate that the researchers didn't collect stool samples during this intervention (or maybe they did and are holding for a future paper. Let's hope so). I do like the *Prevotella* connection, as it doesn't discriminate between the vegans/vegetarians and the omnivores, though the *Prevotella* group sample size was small, it was also informative.

For what it's worth, our Mr. B above - the American Gut participant who had levels of *Prevotella* around 32% - also took a week of broad-spectrum antibiotics. And for giggles, he submitted another stool sample at the end of the antibiotic course. Interestingly, his levels of *Prevotella* went from 32% down to 13%. Does this mean his 'potential circulating levels of TMAO' would have gone down if they had been measured? Who knows? And maybe the *Prevotella* went down in the antibiotic group above as well, i.e. the group that was unable to produce TMAO after antibiotics.

If enriched levels of *Prevotella* are in fact associated with higher levels of circulating TMAO (and you buy into the current thesis that TMAO accelerates atherosclerosis) then it's worth paying attention to. If elevated levels of *Prevotella* might be associated with whole-grain based diets (but not highly processed carbs), then the genus *Prevotella* has come of age since the advent of agriculture (which is the last 0-10,000 years, more or less, depending on where your ancestors hail from). A potentially interesting question then might be: *is there any deleterious effects associated with the blooming of this genus in our recent evolutionary past?* If humans (and hominids in general) have lived for millions of years with low to no levels of *Prevotella*,

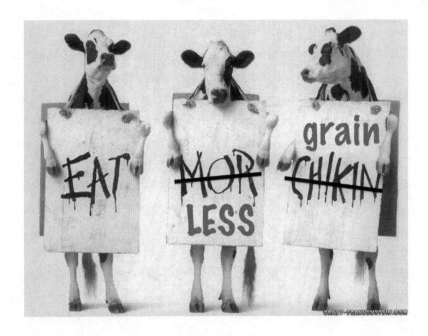

one might suspect that if all of sudden they constituted 30%, 50% or even 90% of the total gut bacteria at any given time in some individuals, then there might be a downside, but nobody knows for sure (as nobody has asked the question). Some *have* suggested they are reservoirs for antibiotic resistant genes (but not all antibiotic genes it appears).

As strange as it may seem by this point in this article, I don't have a horse in this race. In other words, I am not anti-meat nor am I anti-grain. I think if you want to eat meat, knock yourself out. Same goes for breads and pasta - I like those too, I just don't eat them that often. I'm more interested in the microbes and *what they might be trying to tell us*. In the not so distant future (which cannot come soon enough), I predict we will all become proficient 'microbial whisperers' when science hands us the tools while the basics of ecology become core modules in our educational systems - top to bottom. Betwixt the twain, as they say, lies some true understanding of human ecology and thus, optimal human health.

Humans have been eating meat (and thus carnitine) for a very long time. The question is, are the genes necessary for metabolizing carnitine a recent phenomenon or have they always been with us? If there is some *specific* association between *Prevotella* and the genes capable of metabolizing dietary carnitine, then it appears - possibly - to have been ushered in with the agricultural revolution and has no obvious precedent throughout much of our evolutionary past. How ironic would it be if the microbial ability to metabolize dietary carnitine from red meat is linked to whole-grain consumption?! As for my hardcore Paleo eating brothers and sisters, this is the place in the story where you smile. Even IF *Prevotella* is currently serving as a reservoir today, what's to stop other bacteria from taking up the genetic call of duty to metabolize carnitine if *Prevotella* were to somehow get depressed at a population level?

As for the title of the *Nature Medicine* article; *'Intestinal microbiota metabolism of L-carnitine, a nutrient in red meat, promotes atherosclerosis'* - a more appropriate title may have been *'Researchers get vegan to eat steak - sun rises next day.'*

REWILD

Please Pass the Microbes

I RECENTLY ACCOMPANIED TWO HADZA HUNTERS to a series of seeps (or springs) where they had set up hunting blinds of tall grass to ambush thirsty animals. It's late dry season here in Tanzania and dwindling water sources force otherwise dispersed animals to aggregate (and if you're a hunter-gatherer, this is a good thing). The previous week a hunter killed a zebra from one of these blinds with a poison tipped arrow and a windfall of >400-500 pounds of protein and fat that would be consumed in <72 hours. On our way back to camp we came across another Hadza, who had only moments before killed an adult impala. After helping hoist the deceased into a low-hanging tree, letting it hang by its head for field dressing, I witnessed something which made me realize that up until that point, I had not fully appreciated the significance around the co-evolution of human beings, our microbes and the potentially profound implications for our health in the modern world.

I had come to Tanzania as part of a collaboration of U.S, Canadian and Tanzanian researchers to try and understand what the gut microbiome might look like in a group that still hunts and forages 95-100% of its food and more interestingly, how pronounced seasonal changes in resources - e.g. between wet and dry seasons - might impact compositional and functional changes in the microbiota. One pressing question in microbiome research (at least what the public and many public health officials want to know (not to mention food manufacturers and Big Pharma)), is, *"Is there an optimal composition of gut microbes we should strive for and at what age, and what diet and lifestyle choices will get us to this microbial fountain of health?"* This is, of course, a rather complex question.

The Hadza may provide some interesting insight into this question as they live in a part of Africa that presumably gave rise to our genus (*Homo*) and our more distant tree-hugging ancestors. The Hadza still hunt and forage many of the animals and plants that our ancestors relied upon. They are covered in the same soil, drink the same water and follow more or less a seasonal, hunter-gatherer lifestyle that dominated the last two million plus years of human evolution. While it's important to understand how humans lived once they left Africa and settled other parts of the planet in the last ~60,000 years, the huge spans of time our kind spent in Africa, evolving towards the lion's share of our current physiology (as well as our current adaptive immunity), is potentially even more interesting when it comes to understanding the human-microbe relationship - both good and bad.

Importantly, the Hadza don't keep livestock or plant foods of any kind and have limited access to modern medications like antibiotics (at least this is the case for the more

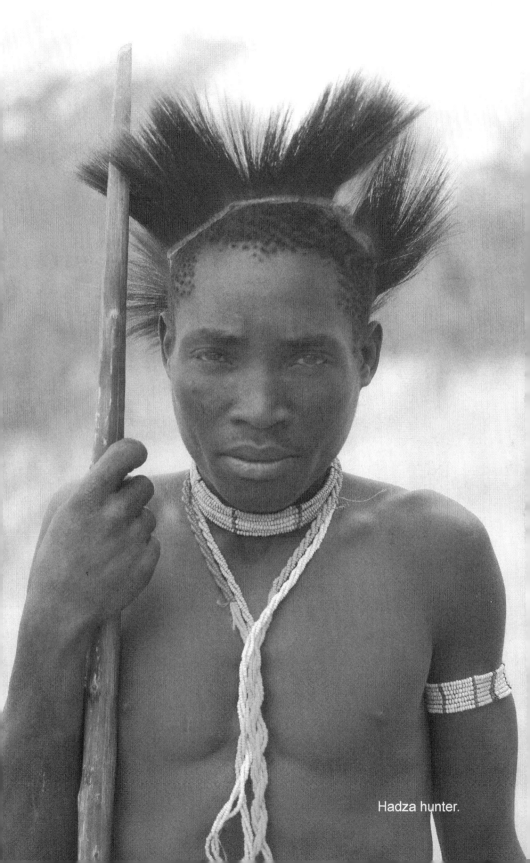

Hadza hunter.

remote Hadza camps we are studying). While some may argue that the Hadza are not perfect referents for 'the way it once was,' it really depends on the questions you are asking. For our purposes, studying how humans acquire microbes from birth throughout life (from others and the larger meta community of microbes in nature), in a group where babies are all still born naturally (no cesarean sections) - and who are breastfed on average for 2+ years, where children still sleep with their mothers years beyond weaning, take no antibiotics, never drink water that has been treated with chlorine and fluoride, where multiple generations stay together (not separating the seniors into assisted living facilities), who don't eat processed foods and where newborns through to the eldest in the community are still covered in nature's blanket of everything that comes from living outside 24/7 and interacting in an intimate way with 100's of species of plants and animals, well they fitted our prerequisites perfectly.

Back to the impala.

Before the two Hadza men jumped in to help skin and gut the impala, I quickly took swabs of each of their hands (after 1 hour, 3 hours and so on) to assess how the skin of the palm microbiota changed throughout the day/week of a typical Hadza. (We've sampled the hands and stools of 300 + Hadza men, women and children so far). As they slowly and methodically dismembered the animal, they carefully placed the stomach and it's still steaming contents onto the fleshy side of the recently removed hide. In a separate area, they piled the fatty internal organs (which men are only allowed to eat, by the way). Once the animal had been processed more or less, I was amazed to see all three men take a handful of the partially

34

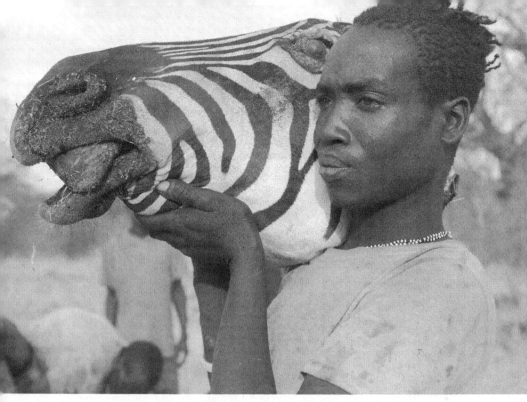

Hadza man and the head of a recently dispatched zebra shot with a poison-tipped arrow.

digested plant material from the recently removed stomach to scrub off the copious amounts of blood that now covered their hands and forearms. This was followed by a final 'cleaning' with dry grass for good measure.

While I was fascinated by the microbe-laden stomach contents being used as hand scrubber (presumably transferring an extraordinary diversity of microbes from the impala gut to the hands of the Hadza), I was not at all prepared for what they did next. Once they had cleaned out - by hand - the contents of the stomach ('cleaned' is actually a generous word), they carved pieces of the stomach into bite-sized chunks and consumed it - 'sushi-style'. By 'sushi-style' I mean that they didn't cook it or even attempt to kill or eliminate the microbes from the gut of the impala in anyway and if this unprecedented transfer of microbes from the skin, blood and stomach of another mammal wasn't enough, they then turned their attention to the colon of the Impala.

After removing the poo pellets (which we collect samples of as well), they tossed the tubular colon onto a hastily built fire. It sat on the fire for a minute at best (clearly not long enough to terminate the menagerie of invisible microbes clinging to the inside wall of the colon) and then proceeded to cut the colon into chunks and to eat it more or less raw. I kindly turned down offers to taste both the raw stomach and the partially cooked colon but I did eat some tasty impala ribs that I thoroughly turned on a stick over the fire to a microbial-free state of 'well done'.

The Hadza explained that this is what they always do and what they have always done (though I suspect the sushi-style eating of innards is not an every-kill ritual). So whether it's an impala, dik dik, zebra, bush pig, kudu or any other of the myriad of mammals they hunt and eat, *becoming one* with the deceased's microbes in any number of ways is simply common place, and same goes for 700 plus species of birds they hunt (minus the abundant amounts of stomach contents for hand sanitizer). In a much less obvious way than at the 'kill site,' the transfer of microbes continued back in camp when the women, children and other men handled the newly arrived raw meat, internal organs and skin. The transfer continued as the hunters engaged (i.e. touching) other members of the camp.

The breathtaking exchange that is the 'horizontal transfer' of microbes between the Hadza and their environment is more or less how it's been for eons, until humans started walling ourselves off from the microbial world through the many facets of globalization. Rather than think of ourselves as isolated islands of microbes, the Hadza teach us that we are better thought of as an archipelago of islands, once seamlessly

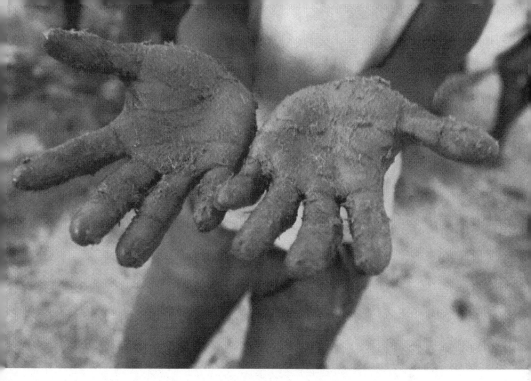

The hands of a Hadza hunter after butchering an animal. Note the microbial-rich stomach contents on his hands.

connected to one another and to a larger metacommunity of microbes via a microbial super highway that runs through the gut and skin/feathers of every animal and water source in the landscape. (For those of you keeping up with your homework, this is Macroecology 101). The same can be said for plants and their extraordinary diversity of microbes above (phyllosphere) and below ground (rhizosphere) that the Hadza (and all humans) once interacted with on a nearly continuous basis.

The Hygiene Hypothesis - or Old Friends Hypothesis, if you prefer - posits that a great many diseases (specifically autoimmune diseases) result from a disconnect with the natural world and its myriad of microscopic life, microbes and other tiny things that once trained our immune system to distinguish between friend or foe (and even the Self). Our children are no longer born in the microbe-rich dirt, but rather hyper-sterile rooms where even the air is scrubbed with mechanical systems. Furthermore, an increasing number of babies are born through an incision rather than the microbial-rich birth canal and the percentage that are still consuming microbial-rich milk from mom at 2 or even 1 year of age can be counted in the low single digits, depending on where you live and your lot in life. Most of our kids (and our adults too, for that matter), have no interaction with extensive microbial networks that the Hadza and our ancestors once experienced. For us, the microbial super highway that once connected all humans to the larger metacommunity of microbes now 'dead ends' at closed windows with very few species of plants in the yard and no (or few) animals except maybe a dog (or two) and a wet wipe or anti microbial something or other at every given turn.

There is no arguing that our modern lifestyle and wonders of modern hygiene, sanitation and medicine have saved a great many lives over previous generations, especially among the youngest in our ranks who are especially vulnerable to diarrheal and respiratory disease (which is still a problem in densely crowded conditions in many developing countries). But as we tout the triumph of the modern lifespan over the 'crueler, harsher life' of the days of yore, we need to keep in mind that our point of reference is the filth and pestilence of the crowded towns and cities of the last millennia or so and *not* the nomadic lifestyle that dominated 99% of human/hominin evolution before we plowed the ground and pinned select animals. Yes, it is true that ~20% of Hadza children die young, but those that survive to adulthood have a good chance to live into their 60's, 70's and 80's. To suggest that we cannot learn about the very foundations of human-microbe mutualism, commensalism, vertical/horizontal transmission and microbial succession across an age gradient in a society unencumbered by the confounders of so-called 'modern life.' childhood mortality rates are seen as extreme medical standards, is to throw the baby out with the bath The Hadza (and the very limited number of groups like them) are disappearing fast and sadly, this potential microbial Noah's Ark will soon be lost.

What we might learn from the Hadza's intimate participation in the microbial super highway (that is the natural world) is made more interesting when you consider a series of experiments recently published in the prestigious journal, *Science*[37]. In an elegant set of experiments, the researchers took stool samples from several sets of twins discordant for obesity and inserted them into germ-free mice. In other words, one of the twins was lean while the other was a little chunky. As with previous experiments, the transplanting poo from the obese twin made the recipient mice obese and the poo from the leaner twin resulted in lean mice, demonstrating that host phenotype (obese or lean) is transmissible. (I admittedly just glossed over this very detailed study with its many interesting moving parts. If you have access to this journal, I would highly recommend reading the entire paper. That said, one aspect of the study is worth drawing additional attention (which also happens to be the part of the multi-faceted study that received the most attention from the media).

After taking germ-free mice and inoculating them with the microbiota from the lean or chunky twin (thus making the bugged mice fat or lean), they then stuck the lean and fat mice together in the same cage and fed them the exact same diet. Since mice are coprophagic i.e. they eat poo, the researchers were curious to see what happened. Throughout the cohousing of the two groups of mice, the researchers collected fecal samples (careful to keep separate which pellets came from

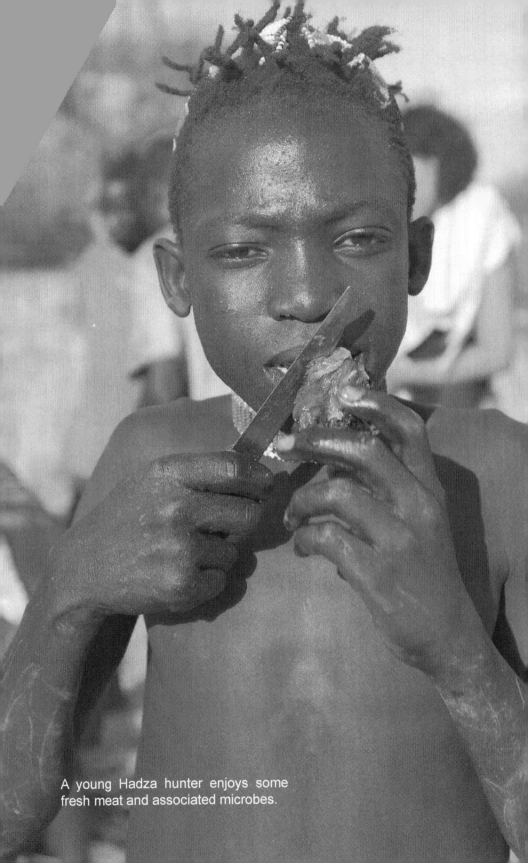

A young Hadza hunter enjoys some fresh meat and associated microbes.

which mouse) every day more or less for a few weeks whilst monitoring their body composition.

Remarkably, analysis of fresh poo pellets from the mice revealed that several species of bacteria from the lean mice successfully invaded the gut of the fat mice but not the other way around - remember, the mice were eating each other's poo and thus each others microbes. In other words, the gut microbiota of the fat mice reconfigured to look more similar to the lean mice yet, as mentioned, the lean mice microbiota remained stable and did not uptake any bacteria from the obese mice despite eating the fat mice poo. Furthermore, the invasion of species from the lean mice into the obese mice essentially shut down further weight gain in the obese mice. Interesting also to note is that the diet was low fat, high plant polysaccharide and fed *ad libitum* i.e. all you can eat.

Using a snazzy piece of analytical wizardry, the researchers were able to track exactly which species had successfully invaded the gut of the obese mice from eating the poo of the lean mice. Of the handful of species that invaded the gut of the obese mice from their lean cage mates, *Bacteroides* spp. from the phylum *Bacteroidetes* were largely responsible in protecting against increased adiposity in the fat mice.

Since it appeared that various *Bacteroides* spp. were not only successful invaders but also conferred some kind of leanness, the researchers cooked up a cocktail of a number of *Bacteroides* spp. and a handful of others (39 species in all) and did the experiment all over again. This time they put obese mice (made obese from the chunky twin's microbiota) in a cage and cohoused them with originally germ-free mice that received only the cocktail of 39 species. This time around, the lean mice poo of the 39 specific species was unable to protect the obese mice from getting chunkier. This experiment demonstrated that its not one strain or handful of strains that confer less adiposity and more leanness in obese mice, but that it's more complex interactions which underlie the protection against adiposity.

In one final experiment, they put mice inoculated with the full microbiota from a lean and obese human twin and stuck them in the same cage. The result was the same as before however this time they changed the diet to high saturated fat, low fruit and vegetable i.e. low fiber. Like the previous experiment, the mice consumed one another's poo, but this time the bacteria from the lean mice didn't successfully invade the gut of the obese mice. This suggests the underlying mechanism for protection from obesity (in this particular experiment) is more complex, possibly involving a great many more community members than just a handful of species and just a handful of species with diet playing a major role.

In the context of the experiments discussed in the *Science* paper, I can't help but think that us modern folk moving through our squeaky clean lives - obsessing over every bite of food we eat - might be suffering (oh so slightly) from a detour (or full blown exit) from the microbial super highway that once dominated so much of our evolutionary history. Though the Hadza (and presumably our ancestors) didn't directly consume each other feces or that of the animals in the landscape on a frequent basis, clearly our hunter-gatherer ancestors had much more of an intimate involvement in the total microbial metacommunity of the environments they inhabited than what we do in the concrete jungles we've come to call 'home.'

Considering this microbial web, it's simply impossible to believe that our ancestors *didn't* benefit in some way with the nearly daily samplings and exchanges of microbes via animals as diverse as zebra, impala, birds and even carnivores like lions (which the Hadza eat by the way), or from the dizzying number of plants sprouting from soil teeming with bacteria (and their genes)). Not only is this benefit plausible - it's highly likely.

Sorry low carbers, your microbiome is just not that into you.

I RECENTLY POSTED A SCATTER PLOT ON SOCIAL media of preliminary metadata that we are accumulating as part of the American Gut project, which includes, among other things, a questionnaire of 50+ questions as well as a seven-day food journal (recently this has been changed to a simple food questionaire). Plotting participants self-reported height, weight and seven days of dietary info - which was recorded using an online calorie counter. We plotted the percentage of daily calories from fat (all sources) against the participant's body mass index (BMI), which we calculated from the height and weight of the participant. While the data is of the dreaded 'self-reported' kind, the *lack of any significant correlation* between the percentage of daily calories from fat and BMI is still very interesting. Note even if you remove the various obvious outliers, the correlation (or lack of) is the same.

In other words, as fat goes up in the diet, BMI does not *per se*.

As I look at the preliminary generic metadata and follow the conversation around the benefits of a low carb diet, I continue to be concerned about the low-carbers gut microbiota. I eat meat daily so my diet is high in fat and animal protein but I also consume dietary fiber from a large diversity and quantity of plants (and I don't consume many grains in any form). While there is no denying the wonderful results many people enjoy on a low (and even lower) carb diet - specifically weight loss, which is well-documented now in the peer-review research - *the impact on the gut microbiota is still not well understood*. As we can see from our accumulating metadata (with an ultimate goal of 20,000 participants (we are at 6,000 now) with complete metadata on ~1,000 so far), we are likely (and hopeful) to have a decent sample of low carb dieters. This data will allow us to compare the gut microbial communities of this population against other dietary strategies. Again, please note we have not completed sequencing of the very low, low carb eaters and so are not presenting any of that data. The plot is just metadata on fat and BMI, which tells us nothing about gut health of the various dots in the plot. The following discussion is based on some general observations based on the existing literature about fermentation, pH and its impact on the gut microbiome.

Depending on whom you talk with, a low carb diet is many different things to many people. I think most misinterpret a Paleo or Primal lifestyle as somehow low carb. It can be, but most folks eat a diversity and quantity of whole plants that exceed that of the average American, often by a long shot. It can sometimes be a little low carb-*like* due to the absence of high caloric foods made from grains, yet I often find people who skip grains, sugar and the like as really paying attention to whole plants in their diet, which is, of course, a good thing. A *bona fide* low, low carb eater is another animal altogether. Whether you draw that line at a carb intake of 25g, 50g or 75g a day, I'm afraid it's low from the perspective of your gut bugs, especially if those carbs contain a limited amount of resistant starch and other dietary fibers - all food for gut bacteria.

That said, even though someone who eats as much as 200-500g of carbs a day can still be starving their guts bugs (if those foods contain little to no indigestible substrates (fiber)). A generic rule of thumb (albeit an ugly measure) is less *overall* carbohydrates, especially when you start dropping below 75-100g a day. This then translates into a dramatic drop in the amount of food reaching your colon where the vast majority of your intestinal microbial community resides.

There are exceptions to every rule, but follow my logic for a moment: when it comes to the health and well being of your gut microbes, nothing matters more than fermentable substrates[26]. As the rules & tenants of basic microbial ecology go, a reduction in fermentable substrates (derived from carbohydrates) means less energy sources for the microbes[27] who depend on host-derived substrates as well, as in the case of mucin-degraders like Akkermansia[28]. As fermentation drops, so to does the byproducts of fermentation, which include short chain fatty acids (primarily acetate, butyrate and propionate), organic acids, and gases like hydrogen. All of this can *(and will)* dramatically shift the pH of the colonic environment. As it stands in a healthy, normal gut, the pH of the colon changes from proximal to distal[29] end, being more acidic in the proximal (front) end than the tail end, mainly as a function of more rapid fermentation as food items empty from the small intestine. As the pH shifts to being more alkaline from less fermentation, a number of shoes begin to drop (or can).

A less acidic environment means acid sensitive groups of bacteria (like those in the Phylum Proteobacteria, a who's who of 'bad guys' such as E. Coli, Salmonella, Vibrio, Helicobacter) *might* bloom, which is not a good thing. You see the same 'blooms' following antibiotic treatment[30]. In addition, as pH shifts away from acidic[31], the genus *Bacteroides* can also bloom, gaining an ecological niche in this less acidic environment, courtesy of a low carb diet. For those of you keeping score, many talk about the American gut in general being dominated by *Bacteroides* as a function of our high fat, high sugar diet. The reality is, it *might* have to do with what we are *not* eating i.e. dietary fiber (of all kinds). The all-important butyrate producers; Roseburia spp. & Eubacterium, also drop in abundance as pH shifts away from acidic. A drop in fecal butyrate and butyrate producing bacteria was demonstrated in an elegant study[32] comparing diets consisting of varying amounts of carbs. Given the importance of butyrate in colonic health, any dietary strategy that potentially shifts pH *away* from acidity as a function of reduced fermentation might contribute to various forms of IBD[33].

Low carb therefore equals a less acidic colonic environment due to the drop in fermentation (and I presume harder and less frequent stools as a function of reduced biomass from bacteria - or maybe not). As pH shifts, prospects for opportunistic pathogens increase, as do opportunities for gram-negative bacteria like *Bacteroides* & Enterobacter. When you add this up while addressing the many other shifts in the microbial ecology of the low carb gut, you most certainly have a classic case of *microbial dysbiosis* which is, as the name implies, an *imbalance*. This dysbiosis[34] can then lead to issues associated with IBD, autoimmune disease, metabolic disorders and so on but again, a large cohort of the low, low carb dieters have never been looked at using 16S rRNA methods, so the jury is still out and the results will be fascinating to see.

The minor paradox in all of this is the increased likelihood that a low carb microbial community will most certainly lead to increased gut permeability, a well-known phenomenon[35] whereby microbial parts (excess lipopolysaccharides, which lead to metabolic endotoxemia[36]) and whole microbes themselves (*bacteremia*) leak from the intestinal tract into the blood, leading to low-grade inflammation that is at the root of metabolic diseases such as type 2 diabetes, obesity and heart disease. It is a paradox that a leaky gut can be triggered from a low carb (high fat) diet, but that a possible increase in gram-negative bacteria and a reduction in healthy bacteria like *Bifidobacterium* does *not* result in weight gain (as demonstrated in study after study in mice and humans). Weird.

I hope people do not take this as some kind of attack on low carb diets. That couldn't be further from the truth. There is NO AGENDA I repeat, NO AGENDA (and it's worth noting again that I consume a high fat, high protein, high fiber diet). I just wanted to point out some obvious concerns (perhaps unfounded), and that if we get a large enough sample of low carb folks in The American Gut Project, we might be able to provide some interesting insight - or we might not - so who knows, maybe low carb folks have super healthy gut microbiota (whatever *that* is).

In closing, I'd like to say to all my low carb brothers and sisters out there, try and eat a little more fibrous material if you can. Diversity matters, and helping your gut bugs definitely helps you because after all, it's what evolution intended.

REWILD

Going Feral: my one-year journey to acquire the healthiest gut microbiome in the world (you heard me!)

UNLESS YOU'VE BEEN HOLED UP IN A CABIN IN the Siberian outback, it's been hard to miss the avalanche of research and associated press coverage ballyhooing the connection between microbes and human health and disease in 2015. 2016 will be no different, as fecal transplants become the new black.

Name just about any ailment plaguing humanity and you will find some researcher somewhere, working the *microbial angle* for a causal or correlative connection. More federal funding please!

Reading between the lines of the near breathless and optimistic reporting on the human microbiome sits a sobering fact: scientists know very little about the connection between disease and the potential microbial culprits (these are very early days). Science is hard and the human gut is a vast and diverse ecosystem. As with any ecosystem, it's the community as a whole that's likely more important and not single members *per se*. Connecting the dots when there are lots of them - dots that are shape shifting all the time - is proving to be tough (as well as slowing our understanding of the role of human genes in disease). This will take some time but the writing's on the wall.

That said, projects like American Gut are trying to map the diversity of the human gut. By sequencing the gut microbes of tens of thousands of regular folks of all shapes, sizes and of diverse diet and lifestyles, we hope to see coarse-grained patterns shaped by disease, state, age, diet, lifestyle habits and so on. These broad strokes will then allow researchers from all over the world (yes, de-identified American Gut data is open source and made available to the research community thanks to the good folks over at Earth Microbiome Project[38]) to dig a little deeper to see what might matter the most when it comes to maintaining a healthy microbiome at different stages of life and yup, a 2 year old harbors very different microbial compositions than their grandpa.

In addition to a large sample of westerners, we will also be able to compare these tens of thousands of samples to other data sets, including groups from Africa, India, South America and so on. Excitingly, our work with the Hadza hunter-gatherers in Tanzania will allow us to compare our western selves to people who still hunt and gather the majority of their food, have limited access to western medications, are all born naturally and breastfed for 2+ years, live outside more or less 24/7, are covered in microbial-laden soil (nature's blanket) and that have an intimate connection to a vast (natural) microbial world that we in the so-called developed world have moved away from. We don't know what we will learn over the coming years but it is a given that we will be a little smarter when it comes to modulating and nudging our gut microbes in a healthier direction with diet and lifestyle choices (and I sure hate to see Big Pharma drug our microbiome into compliance so lets not let it happen folks!).

As researchers continue to build the scientific case for the microbe-health connection in 2015, I'm embarking on a little self-exploration. Beginning on January 1st 2014, I began the first of many different 'diets' that I hope will lead to a better understanding (at least for me), of not only what a healthier gut microbiome might look like in a modern world, but also more importantly; what it *shouldn't* look like. I will be collecting daily stool samples along the way for subsequent 16S rRNA analysis over the next 365 days.

On January 1st I started a high fat, protein diet with very, very little carbohydrates and near zero quantities of dietary fiber. In short, I'm attempting to starve my microbes of much-needed substrates for growth such as dietary fiber, resistant starch etc. I'm not arguing that anyone should do this on a regular basis, nor am I suggesting this is a good or bad dietary strategy, but I am trying to whack my microbiome around a bit to demonstrate that significant shifts in your gut microbiota can be achieved in very short periods of time with significant shifts in macronutrients.

I experienced this past summer how dramatically you can shift your gut bugs with diet when I traveled from New Orleans to West Texas where I was held up for a few months trying to finish a book (*BLOOM*; forthcoming, Victory Publishing). As I drove out of New Orleans I left behind a diet heavy on meat but with a quantity and diversity of dietary fiber that would make Michelle Obama smile. Once I landed in the parched landscape of West Texas near Big Bend National Park and arrived at the little writers shack I rented, I saw that the

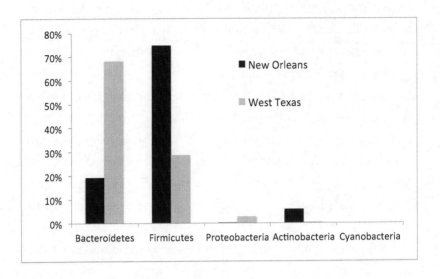

dwelling lacked some modern niceties, such as a kitchen. Consequentially, I ate most of my meals at the local watering holes. Below is a graph of what happened to my gut microbes.

As the graph above reveals, I look like an entirely different person 'microbially-speaking.' My New Orleans microbiome were dominated by the phyla Firmicutes (74.80%) but after only 2-3 weeks of greatly reduced consumption of dietary fiber - and remember, I still ate lots of meat - my Firmicutes dropped to 28.63% while my Bacteroidetes shot up. In other words, my Firmicutes and Bacteroidetes traded places in my new desert belly.

Digging a little deeper in the data reveals that much of this dramatic shift can be attributed to a handful of genera. My *Bacteroides* (in the phyla Bacteroidetes) seem to really like my zero to super low plant intake, going from a mere 15.91% relative abundance in New Orleans to a whopping 56.59% in my near plantless desert diet. Consequently, the relative abundance of the Family *Ruminococcaceae* took a hit along with the Family *Lachnospiraceae* and the Genus *Ruminococcus*. These three are known plant fermenters (i.e. they metabolize dietary plant polysaccharides), that didn't seem to compete very well as the fermentable substrates (fiber and resistant starch) dried up.

Also of interest are my *Bifidobacterium* levels, which went from 5.46% in New Orleans, to 0.10% and my levels of Paraprevotella (kissing cousin of *Prevotella*) went from a paltry 0.40% to a monstrous 7.20% in the desert. In the case of *Bifidobacterium* levels taking a hit (and please note that I like *Bifidobacterium* as they are often cited as being part of a healthy and balanced gut flora), I would go out on a limb and suggest they were suppressed due to my lack of onions, garlic, leek etc. and though I suspect I could be wrong, that's my hunch at the moment.

As for the increase *Paraprevotella*, I would again go out on a limb and suggest this spike is attributed to my modest intake of whole grains via muesli-like cereal, essentially eaten dry every morning in my desert home and something I didn't do in New Orleans. Anyone that follows the Human Food Project blog knows I have something of a *(Para)Prevotella* fetish and attribute the increased relative abundance in folk as a sign of 'whole' grain consumption, not fiber intake *per se* as often argued[39]. Strikingly, elevated levels of *Prevotella* have been noted among HIV-infected individuals who exhibit chronic gut inflammation. In this study[40], the researchers suggest that *Prevotella* may thrive under conditions of inflammation.

In another study[41], researchers found that *Prevotella* strongly correlated with new-onset untreated rheumatoid arthritis. On the flipside, reduced rather than increased levels of *Prevotella* correlated with kids diagnosed with autism compared to symptom-free neurotypical children in a recent study[42]. It's also interesting to note that many families will place ASD kids on a gluten and casein free diet following diagnosis. Therefore, if my 'out on a limb' theory that *Prevotella* levels are associated with whole grain consumption is near the mark, then lower levels of *Prevotella* in these diagnosed youngsters is not completely unexpected. In other words, in diagnosed ASD kids the lower to zero levels of *Prevotella* may have more to do with diet than the disease state, but we will wait and see how this shakes out over the coming years.

If you spend anytime reading the literature on *Bacteroides* - the genus that dominated my desert belly - you will quickly surmise that most researchers attribute it to a high-fat western diet. During my little New Orleans to desert diet experiment my levels of meat and thus, by extension, my levels of fat and protein - stayed more or less the same. The only thing that substantially changed was my reduction in plants and the fermentable fibers they contain, so in my Sample Size of One, changes in my intake of meat can't really explain the striking shifts seen in the graphs above. Perhaps rather than *Bacteroides* 'thriving in a fat-soaked environment of my desert gut,' they likely gained a toehold in my increasingly alkaline gut. Like many microbes, many strains of *Bacteroides* seem to be pH sensitive[43], and the main driver of the acidity of your colon is *fermentation*. Reduce the amount of dietary fiber and resistant starch reaching your colon (i.e. no plants), and pH will rise, becoming more alkaline due to a reduction of short chain fatty acids and other organic acids that are byproducts produced during fermentation. As pH rises, the microbes that are otherwise pH sensitive tend to bloom. Therefore, my 'out on a limb' interpretation of the dramatic shift in my microbial community in the example/experiment above is not driven by increased meat consumption, but rather my shift in pH due to the *lack of fermentation*, which ultimately provided fertile ground for *Bacteroides* to dominate.

My increase in the phyla Proteobacteria from 0.03% in New Orleans to 2.63% in the desert suggests that this new, less acidic ecosystem may have favored some opportunistic pathogens. One final gut check (the most concerning of all to me), showed that the overall diversity of my gut microbiota was halved in the desert (as measured by species equivalent OTU's), and so as Ecosystems 101 teaches us, a less diverse microbiota[44] is *less resilient* to perturbations and may tip one a tad closer to an unhealthy state. One recent study[45] suggests that my reduction in gut microbial diversity - while not dramatically altering my sanitation and hygiene practices in the process - may have had a lot to do with my reduction in dietary fiber. This has also been seen in mice fed high versus low fiber diets (personal communication, Justin Sonnenburg, Stanford University).

It's my little experiment, coupled with a steady flow of papers suggesting diet and lifestyle can dramatically impact your gut microbial composition in short period of time[46], that has led me to my 2014 goal of acquiring and *catching* the healthiest gut microbiome in the world. By *catching*, I mean it's not *all* about what you eat, but *how and where you live* - and whom you live with - as well as your interaction with the microbial world around us.

Throughout 2015 I will undertake a series of dramatic shifts in my diet and lifestyle in an attempt to whack my microbiome around. For example, aside from the high fat/ protein diet I finished at the start of the year (taking poo samples along the way), I will go on a raw food diet for a few weeks, followed by a juicing diet, (possibly followed by a vegan diet), followed by an Atkins-like diet, followed by a Mediterranean diet, followed by a period of fasting. This will all be (possibly) followed by weeks of fermented foods, a Paleo diet, Jenny Craig and Weight Watchers diets, a Master Cleanse Diet and so forth. Some of these diets will be repeated several times. I will also go on the occasional drinking binge, exploring the impact of beer, wine and Jose Cuervo on my microbiota. Don't tell anyone, but I will also explore the impact of copious amounts of weed as I wake and bake for a week while holding various diets constant. Perhaps the most interesting will be the hunter-gatherer plunge I will take 2-3 times as I live and work among the Hadza hunter-gatherers of Tanzania where I started working in 2013 (*Science*[47] did a nice three-pager on our project recently if you want to learn more - see also the tiny blurb in *Nature*[48]). As a newly minted hunter-gatherer I will live in a grass hut, forage for plants and consume wild game (zebra, impala, kudu, baboons, warthog, birds etc.) and drink their water, all the while collecting my stool samples. It will be interesting to see if I can shift my western gut - whichever one I have at the time - to look more like the Hadza. I suspect my exposure to the microbes in the Hadza environment will dramatically alter my microbial composition and increase the overall diversity, but the question is; *will it last when I return home?*

I'm not sure what I will learn at this point, but I will share my results with colleagues and ask them to weigh in on the microbial compositions generated by the various diets. I will also ask them to do so without them having any knowledge of the diet that produced the results in an effort to remove bias against any particular diet/strategy/lifestyle, such as the bias we see over at US News & World Report[49] as they continue to deliver an annual ass-whopping to the Paleo diet, as they rank the healthiest diet on an annual basis. Will I nail down the diet and lifestyle that results in an optimal microbiome, whatever that is? I really don't know for sure but I'm pretty confident I will learn which diet and lifestyle choices yield less than optimal outcomes for my gut bugs. If anyone out there has any diets - crazy or mainstream - that they would like me to consider, drop me a note - and let the games begin.

(Re)Becoming Human

AS THE SUN SET OVER LAKE EYASI IN TANZANIA, nearly thirty minutes had passed since I had inserted a turkey baster into my bum and injected the feces of a Hadza man - a member of one of the last remaining hunter-gatherers tribes in the world - into the nether regions of my distal colon. I struggled to keep my legs in the air with my toes pointing towards what I thought was the faint outline of the Southern Cross rising in the evening sky. With my hands under my hips and butt perched against a large rock for support, I peddled an imaginary upside down bicycle in the air to pass the time as I struggled to make sure my new gut ecosystem stayed put inside me.

With my butt cheeks flexed and my 'you know what' puckered, I wondered if I had just made a terrible, terrible mistake. Could I really displace my western gut microbial ecosystem with that of a man who only days before had dined on animals as diverse as zebra and monkey and who possessed one of the most diverse gut microbiomes of any person on the planet? Would my immune system soon freak out at the presence of what should be some familiar, old (microbial) friends now setting up shop throughout the slimy vastness of my gastrointestinal tract or had I just unwittingly infected myself with some lethal bacteria or virus? The pros and cons - mostly cons - of my turkey basting activities raced through my anxious mind as I peddled my way into the evening.

My colleagues and I have been working and living amongst the Hadza hunter-gatherers of Tanzania for over a year now. Over the course of several field sessions, we've collected nearly 2000 human and environmental samples in an attempt to characterize the microbes on and within the Hadza as well as the microbes in their environment. The human samples have mostly included stool (feces), but also swabs of hands, foreheads, bottoms of feet, tongues (some spit), breast milk from mothers and so on. Environmental sampling has included swabs of the plants and other foods they consume such as berries, roots, honey etc. in addition to a dizzying number of animals ranging from greater kudu, impala, dik dik, zebra, various monkeys and birds and so on. For the animals, we collect their feces and when possible, swabs of the stomach contents of larger animals, all of which end up covering the Hadza sooner or later during butchering. We also swab their homes inside and out, along with their various water sources. In short, we swab everything, including the researchers while in the field.

The project includes a talented team of collaborators from New York University, University of Colorado-Boulder, Stanford, Mount Sinai School of Medicine, Western University & Lawson Health Research Center in Canada and several

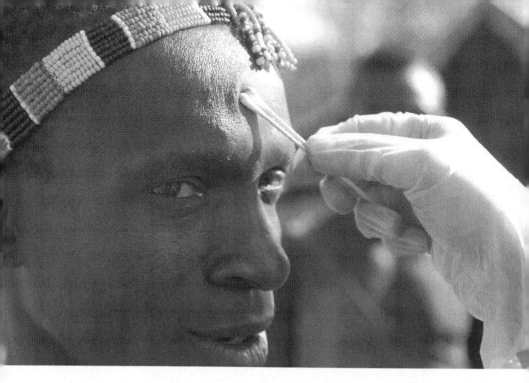

A colleague taking a skin swab from the forehead of a Hadza man. These samples, along with other body sites, will allow us to characterize the skin microbiome of the Hadza.

researchers from the National Institute of Medical Research in Tanzania. Additional collaborators working on various analysis are scattered at universities across the US and Europe.

Among many things, we are interested in how Hadza microbes (along with their environmental microbes such as water, homes, plants and animals), shift between the wet and dry seasons. Due to some unique geography and global weather patterns[50], East Africa experiences a striking wet and dry season - essentially 6 months of on and off rain - followed by almost none. This reality means that during the dry season as the water holes dry up, the Hadza kill a lot more animals (as their dwindling water sources make the animals more predictable and easier to shoot with their poison arrows from hunting blinds aka ambush hunting). An increase in protein and fat from these animals means a drop off in other caloric resources - mainly plants - as the Hadza will often binge on meat when possible. Note they have no storage so everything is eaten in a short period of time. During the wet season when *Hadza Land* is awash in greenery and flowers, the Hadza enjoy an abundance of wild honey (fat of the larvae included) and massive stands of sugary berries. With the coming of the rains, larger animals are more scattered and thus harder to kill so they make up less of the daily calories, though it's highly variable from day-to-day and week-to-week and from camp-to-camp. No matter the season, fibrous baobab fruit and subsurface tubers are a daily constant for the Hadza. Yes, they consume lots and lots of dietary fiber.

The impact of seasonality on the Hadza and their microbial environment is an interesting and possibly very important question as it relates to what a healthier microbiome *might* have looked like - before the comforts and medications of the current modern era whacked the crap out of our gut bugs. It's not a stretch to say that nearly all of us in the western world are a hot microbial mess due to well, just about every aspect of our daily lives. Hence the emerging microbial connection to a staggering number of diseases and ailments in the twenty-first century including IBD, autoimmune diseases, obesity, type 2 diabetes and so on.

Should we *really* strive for a certain composition of gut microbes, as many modern buggy-like products infer, such as those found in over the counter probiotics as well as various other health drinks and foods? Or does the reality of our seasonal past reveal that our gut microbiome is a shape shifting metabolic organ pulling the strings of our health and well being in a bi-annual (or even tri-annual) circadian-like rhythm? Said differently, (and with all due respect to the brilliant Harvard

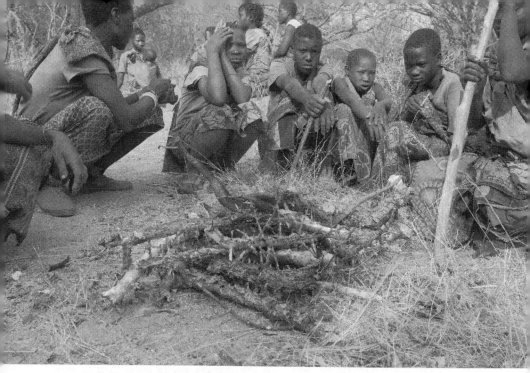

Hadza women lightly cooking recently dug //ekwa roots. Hadza eat fibrious roots on a daily basis.

researcher Richard Wrangham of *fire made us human fame*), *is* seasonality and its impact on our symbiotic microbes more responsible for what makes us human? I like to think it might be, plus *'Seasonal Homo'* is kind of catchy.

The Hadza are particularly (microbially) interesting over say, other remote groups in South America as they still live in a part of Africa that purportedly gave rise to our genus - *Homo*. However, Lee Berger and his colleagues[51] working new fossil sites in South Africa are giving East Africa a run for its money for the prize for deciding 'which part of Africa holds the honor to the geographical cradle of humanity'. Regardless, being only a stone's throw from famous paleontological sites like Olduvai Gorge of Leakey fame, the Hadza literally hunt and gather many of the same animals and plants that humans and our ilk have subsisted on for millions of years - not too mention they are covered in the same dirt, drink the same water (save the occasional cow turd floating about), and practice the same central-based foraging that has brought people together in microbial-sharing camps/communities for the better part of the Pleistocene. It is this foraging lifestyle that has endowed the Hadza with an extraordinary diversity of bacteria and it's the *diversity* they carry that is most fascinating when compared to our less diverse western gut.

While the Hadza are not living fossils, nor do they (in anyway) represent a perfect referent population for early human evolution. Their hunting and foraging lifestyle and constant contact with the natural microbial world; natural births, extended breastfeeding and limited access to western medications, makes them one of the better populations in the world for trying to understand what our ancestral microbes may have once looked like, where we got them and at what point in our life history we acquired them - *before* the rest of us ran gut first into the buzzsaw of globalization. (Note I am aware that 'ancestral microbiome' is a loaded term. I could just as easily say 'natural microbiome' or 'non western/minimally impacted microbiome' etc. Clearly there is no ONE ancestral microbiome. My point is that ancestral equals *diversity,* in the context I use it).

It's also important to point out our project is in no way trying to argue that the Hadza diet or the diet of any minimally westernized population (present or past) is what we should be eating today. We will leave those discussions up to others, as it's not a focus in our research. We are simply interested in how a free-living population that is still intimately connected to nature acquires microbes and potentially most interesting of all; has a greater diversity of microbes compared to western populations.

On the original question of whether or not the gut microbiome composition of the Hadza changes between wet and dry seasons, our initial (yet unpublished data) suggests 'yes.' To our knowledge this is the first study to document this pattern among rural and remote populations. Ecologically speaking, this suggests there may not be one steady state (or equilibrium) for the human gut. It's more a moving target with multiple, steady states.

Though we see seasonal shifts in the composition of the Hadza gut microbes across the same individuals, we are currently trying to determine if there exists any functional shift as well. In other words, even if the members shift around from season to season, are the metabolic capabilities (or ecosystem services) of the entire community conserved between seasons - or do they change as well? We should know this in the very near future.

If we squint for a moment and consider the Hadza, along with the seasonality of our ancestral past and its impact on our shape shifting gut microbiota (as relevant to populations in the western world), then we might need to start rethinking an entire industry of probiotics and the like, which suggest that we need a certain set of bugs in the numerous products now on offer. Since we are on the subject of probiotics, some significant and dominant players on the market today include characters with names like '*bifidobacterium*' and 'lactobacillus'. Interestingly, while the Hadza harbor *Bifidobacterium* and lactobacillus while still breast-feeding; these bugs are essentially absent in Hadza post-weaning (i.e. more or less absent after age 5).

This begs the question: should we *really* consider these groups of bacteria as essential and necessary to human health despite what a multi-billion dollar industry tells us? Clearly, mountains of research suggest these lactic acid bacteria are good for us, but are there other more ancestral groups of bugs that may be more 'in tune' with our seasonal gut (post-weaning)? More importantly, do the persistence of *Bifidobacterium* and similar bugs in our western gut - often (mainly) due to continued consumption of cow's milk, ingestion of some probiotic/prebiotic foods and so on into adult life - nudge out or blunt down other members of our gut ecosystem that would otherwise flourish and provide important ecosystem services? We are currently trying to understand this as we perform various co-occurrence analyses of the Hadza data, so stay tuned.

It's also interesting to note that while the most dominant group of bacteria in the American Gut is the genus Bacteroides[52] by a country mile, this group of bacteria is a minor, minor player in the Hadza gut. It's almost non-existent. The prevailing wisdom[53] is that these bacteria are driven by our high protein-fat and sugary diet. However, I think it has a lot more to do with our absence of dietary fiber and resulting alkaline guts. As my own self-experiments have shown, I can turn my *Bacteroides* up or down with the amount of fiber in my diet, irrespective of the amount of other macronutrients like fat. To me at least, I think the dominance of *Bacteroides* in the western gut has to do with pH levels, which are mainly driven by fermentation of dietary fiber (and fermentation of fiber equals more SCFAs and thus a more acidic colonic environment which strains of *Bacteroides* don't like). So with the average American eating less than 20g of fiber a day (which is pitiful), we are likely lugging around the most alkaline guts in human history which, in turn, is allowing certain species of *Bacteroides* (and some opportunistic pathogens) to flourish. Again, if we squint for a moment and lean on the gut of the

Hadza, then maybe we shouldn't *let Bacteroides* dominant our gut because by doing so, who else is getting nudged out or down and potentially dragging us closer to ill health? Who really knows at this point. It will be exciting to see how this turns out with more data over the coming years. I suspect the Hadza keep *Bacteroides* levels low with their high, daily levels of dietary fiber, which keeps their colonic environment very acidic (but this is more of a hunch than something we know for sure at the moment so 'more data needed'). In addition, the 'high protein-fat and sugary argument' doesn't hold with the Hadza either, as they will often gorge on meat-fat and eat piles of sugary honey for weeks on end during the wet season - and we see no blooms in *Bacteroides* when we sample during these periods. **It's the Fiber, Stupid!**

Some of our initial sequencing data on the Hadza reveal extraordinary diversity of certain groups of bacteria. One that sticks out among many is the genus *Prevotella*. Currently, there are only two described/sequenced species of *Prevotella* derived from the human gut: *P. copri* and *P. stercorea*[54]. Strikingly, the Hadza appear to harbor dozens of species! This is interesting as *Prevotella* have been linked/correlated to enhanced susceptibility to arthritis[55] and other issues such as HIV[56]. So, is the diversity of *Prevotella* species in the ancestral Hadza beneficial, benign or possibly even problematic? It's incredible to think that we all once harbored this diversity of *Prevotella* but have lost it through our western diet and lifestyle. At the moment we don't know what to make of the Hadza diversity of this important genus, but we are working on it.

Oxalobacter formigenes is another species of bacteria that most of the Hadza carry and that the rest of us in the western world have more or less lost. Oxalobacter, as an oxalate-degrading gut microbe, has gained attention[57] in recent years

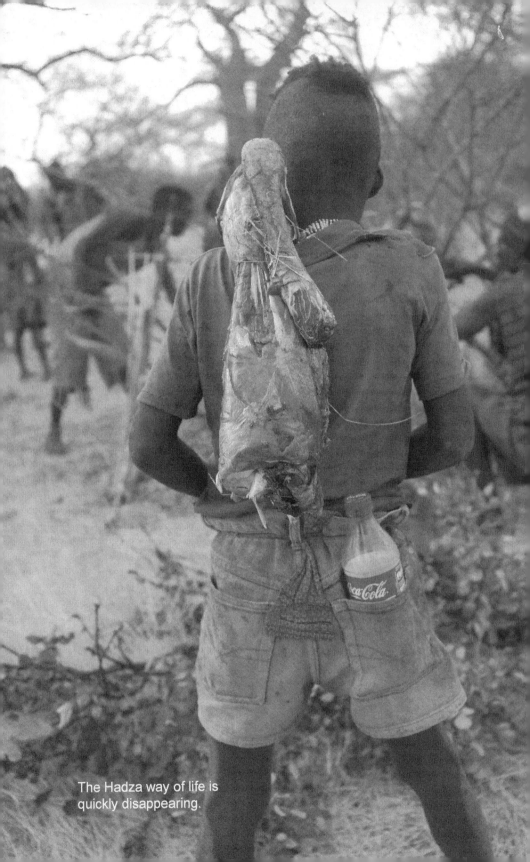

The Hadza way of life is
quickly disappearing.

for its ability for preventing calcium oxalate kidney stones. Graduate students Amanda PeBenito and Lama Nazza in Marty Blaser's lab at NYU have been looking at *Oxalobacter* levels in our Hadza samples and have found that most of the Hadza still carry this important microbe and that they acquire it at a young age. Conversely, *Oxalobacter* seems to be disappearing from our western guts and may be at the root of rising levels of kidney stones. Less than 15% of Americans still carry this important microbe and almost no kids are acquiring it now (according to Amanda and Lama's research). Since Oxalobacter is sensitive to penicillin's, our overuse of some western medications may be the problem.

As the examples of *Prevotella* and *Oxalobacter* reveal – and note there are others emerging in the Hadza samples – we have potentially lost an extraordinary diversity of microbes that may have once contributed to our proper functioning (and the reason I found myself pedaling an imaginary bicycle under a Baobab tree this past August).

During the summer of 2013 when we started working with the Hadza, we would live near them but not in their camps, and though I lived in their environment while working with them, I continued eating western food and collecting my stool samples as well as theirs. Other than the occasional taste of wild meat and some baobab fruit, my diet consisted of pasta, some canned meats, fruits, veggies, booze etc. I was interested in seeing whether or not simply being in their environment would change my gut microbes in any meaningful way. It did – but only slightly. The next field session I not only lived in their environment but drank their water and ate their food – giving up my normal, western camp food. I did smoke weed on occasion, as the Hadza are big pot smokers. (They trade honey and meat for weed with the local Datoga). As with my previous experience, the combination of environment plus Hadza food altered my gut microbe composition. However, my gut bugs still did not match that of an age-matched Hadza male. Granted I did not stay on the Hadza diet long - only 6-8 days at a time. The experiment of 'going Hadza' was to see if I could catch or acquire their consortium of microbes through diet and lifestyle changes. Clearly my changing microbiota suggested 'yes.' Since I did not have the time to live amongst the Hadza for months on end (a time I felt would be necessary to make my gut look more Hadza-like), I thought something a little more radical was required.

Fecal microbiota transplants - FMTs - have become all the rage. As the name implies, it entails taking a small amount of fecal matter from one person and putting into another. While the promise of this therapy is hard to overstate, the science is still a long way down the road from being a simple treatment for everything that ails us in the western world. FMT has been proven again and again as a successful treatment for C. Diff infections (where antibiotics have been unable to clear the infection and in many cases, only make matters worse). FMT use in IBD and other issues is still a work-in-progress but everyone - including me - is hopeful that the idea that you can restore microbial diversity or otherwise improve dysbiosis in a sick gut with a donor stool is really quite breathtaking.

When I first considered the idea of doing a fecal transplant between a Hadza hunter-gatherer and myself, I discussed the idea with a number of colleagues working in various areas of microbiology and medicine as well as others who specialize in fecal transplants. If memory serves, one hundred percent of the experts I consulted told me not to do it. Concerns ran from 'it's too risky' or 'you're not sick so why do it' and so on. It was comical to hear more than a handful of

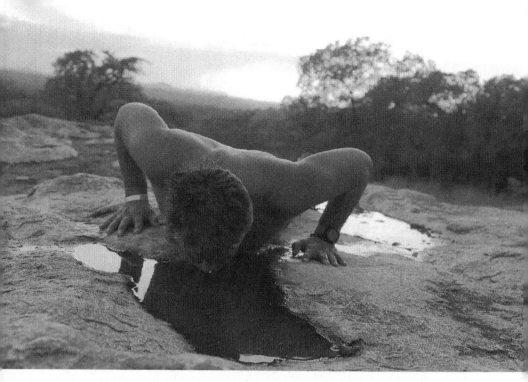

The author on a Hadza diet drinking from a water hole shared by Hadza, baboons, birds and numerous other animals.

experts warn against doing it but also state that if I did, it sure would be interesting to see the data, so I carefully weighed the advice and decided to move forward.

While for ethical reasons I cannot disclose the donor, I can say it was a Hadza male in his mid 30s with a wife and a handful of kids (and the donor provided Informed Consent). Before the poo swap took place, I knew more or less what microbes he carried (as we had sampled him several times over the months prior), and that he harbored at least twice the amount of species (OTUs) that I carried - including all those crazy *Prevotella* and oxalate eating *Oxalobacter*. We also took the donor to a small hospital in the town of Haydom and had him tested for Hepatitis A-C and a few other things. For HIV, we used rapid field test strips and repeated the test multiple times over several days. While it's not possible to catch everything, we were being extremely cautious. However, I had no data on the parasites he might carrying at the time of the transplant as that analysis was still ongoing at the University of Chicago. Oh well, parasites be damned and onward with the science! (Side note: even though parasites get a bad wrap (and rightfully so given that there are some bad guys out there), I am not overly concerned with acquiring them given that they are most likely to play in an important role - past and present - is shaping our gut microbiota).

Since I wasn't sick and in need of a transplant for those reasons - *why was I taking the risk?* To the advice (which I greatly appreciated) from my colleagues, I responded that while I don't technically have a diagnosed disease like a refractory C. diff infection for which a fecal transplant was the best cure, I *did* have a western gut microbiota – one I was given when I passed through my mother's vaginal canal and that I had spent a lifetime of knocking the crap out of with chlorinated tap water, the occasional antibiotic, mountains of shitty (and good) food, living more or less the sterile life of an American male - devoid of the kind of microbes my donor had grown up with - and last but not least, a semi truck load of booze I had consumed as an average American male (I'm 47, so I have seen the bottom of my share of tequila bottles). So I did consider my gut 'sick' even if I had not been diagnosed as such but of course, that's not the whole reason.

The bigger reason or hypothesis I wanted to test was one of *microbial extinction* - something I believe we all suffer from in the western world and may be at the root of what's making us sick. Maria Gloria Dominguez-Bello and Marty Blaser at NYU estimate from their decades of work in the US and among Amerindian populations in South America, that we modern humans have lost a *third* (or more) of the microbial diversity we once enjoyed. The Hadza data thus far suggests that this number could be as high as *half*, so for me and my little transplant experiment with a Hadza hunter-gatherer still living at microbial ground zero for all humans, I wanted to know if my western diet and lifestyle could rapidly destroy this newly acquired diversity in a short period of time. Since the human genome contains ~23,000 genes and our whole-body microbiome accounts for another staggering 5-10 million genes - most of which live deep within our guts - my distal gut ecosystem restoration project attempted to replace 99% of the genes in my body. Said differently, I was not interested in acquiring some exotic microbiome from the donor - and that this would some how be protective for me in the years to come (just by having this different microbiome), but rather I wanted to acquire a large diversity of microbes (which the Hadza carry) so that I could attempt to reduce that diversity, once transitioning back to a western diet and lifestyle. I.e. I'm not really suggesting that the Hadza have a more *ideal* microbiome. We of course do not know this at this point in time, but what we do know is that it's definitely much more diverse).

It has been suggested from several folks that it isn't entirely clear why I did the FMT. Many think it's because I was seeking to acquire a healthier microbiome and thus 'be healthier.' This was NOT the experiment and so, to be clear, the goal was to 1. acquire the diverse microbes from a Hadza and then 2. attempt to WIPE THEM OUT. Yep, the goal was to try and wipe out my newly acquired microbiome. It is the diversity of microbes the Hadza carry in their gut that I'm interested in and the role of diet and lifestyle in reducing that diversity. I've since added/strengthened this point in a number of places in this post where it wasn't sufficiently emphasized.

Again, if you squint with me for a minute, could I simulate 10,000 years of human history - from the transition of hunter-gatherers to agriculturalists, to crowded conditions of civilizations, to indoor plumbing, to the introduction of antibiotics and antimicrobial soaps, to Lady Gaga – all in a short few months with my one fecal transplant?

In all honestly, the things that underlined all of the scientific reasons for doing the transplant and the extraordinary effort it takes to work in East Africa for months on end with the endless stream of setbacks, was my daughter. As anyone who reads the Human Food Project blog on a regular basis knows, she was diagnosed as a type 1 diabetic at ~2 yrs of age - she's 15 now. It is her health issues that drive me everyday to try understand why she acquired such a terrible autoimmune disease. Was it because she was born via c-section and thus skipped the time-honored seeding of microbes from her mother's birth canal? Was it because she was not breast-fed for 2+ years like her ancestors? Was it some medication or the hyper-sterile environment that kids now grow up in the US? Is it because she had a lower diversity of gut microbiota than the ancestors who came before her? I.e. is she a casualty of unintended consequences of the Anthropocene where we all now live? As any parent knows, there is nothing more heart wrenching than watching your child suffer day in and day out with a disease. So yes, I do understand and accept the risks and the many unknowns involved in performing such a fecal transplant with a hunter-gatherer, but in no way does this undermine the emerging importance of fecal transplants for certain ailments and the developing science that underpins it. I do not in anyway take this lightly (nor am I in anyway 'cavalier' about it), but for my daughter & I - and for other families - I feel I have no choice but to do everything I can to try and understand the role of our disappearing microbiota[58] in diseases such as hers. I hope you understand. (And with a sample size of exactly one, I'm aware of the limitations of the SelfExperiment).

So once the fecal transplant had been completed that warm, August night with the aid of a turkey baster (and I'm pretty sure my colleagues who brought me the turkey baster purchased the largest one made and sold at Walmart), I immediately went back to camp and started back on my western diet. Note I had been on a pure Hadza diet for a few days leading up to the transplant.

Before and after the transplant I took stool, blood and urine samples (and I am still taking stool samples weeks after the experiment). We also took several samples of the donor stool. At the writing of this, I'm not sure if the fecal transplant 'took,' i.e. whether my body successfully took the transplant and if it did, what percentage of my donor's bugs populated my distal colon. I was able to 'hold in' the donor's sample until 11AM the next morning - a period of 16 hours - before having my first bowel movement, so I am hopeful. I should know by early November when all the samples are sequenced, whether or not the procedure took.

If I was able to acquire and keep a portion of my donor's ancestral microbial ecosystem, how much of it could I wipe out as I transitioned back to the US and then back to Tanzania this coming Fall? When I arrive back in Tanzania, I will go back on the Hadza diet (and of course, live in their environment) to see how much of the original donor sample I can get to spring back to life. If my transition back to the US results in a loss of my newly acquired diversity, then in essence - if you squint again with me for a moment - I was able to recreate the epidemiological transitions we've all experienced in the last 10,000 years in a few short months. Regardless of the outcome, it will be interesting. I will also do another transplant or two when I return in the Fall, but this time I will stay on the Hadza diet to see if I can hold onto whatever ecosystem I acquire with the transplant.

So how did I feel after the transplant? Not that much different other than - as it was pointed out to me by my girlfriend - I seemed to be farting a LOT less! I didn't really notice any change in my mood (or my bow hunting skills either) but it *is* interesting that I started shedding a few pounds for no apparent reason. Hmm. Stay tuned (and please don't try this at home).

Microbial Diversity: sometimes you have it, sometimes you don't

THIS PAST JANUARY I WANTED TO SEE WHAT would happen to my gut flora if I adopted a hunter-gatherer diet for a week, eating the plants, animals and drinking the same water as the Hadza hunter-gatherers of east Africa (note this was before I performed the fecal transplant described in the previous chapter). Among the other hypothesis I wanted to test: *would immersing myself in this microbial-rich lifestyle increase the diversity of microbes in my tattered western gut?* Below is a PCoA plot of what happened.

Think of a 'PCoA plot' as one of those Christmas snow globes you shake up and then watch the snow sink to the bottom. Since you can turn the globe and watch the snow sink from different angles, it's 3D - and so is the PCoA plot below (though flattened into 2D and viewed from one angle). In short, the closer the dots are together, the more similar the bacteria are in those two or more samples.

The plot on the opposite page shows the timeline of my little experiment. The first three X dots represent my gut bacteria while I was in Arusha, Tanzania in late January of this year. Arusha is a large town just west of Mount Kilimanjaro where the project rents a little house for storing equipment and serves as our base when we are not in the field. While in Arusha I ate some meals at the house, drank the local tap water and ate the occasional meal at a restaurant. Food consists of eggs, bacon, miscellaneous vegetables, chicken and usually a nightcap of whiskey or wine.

Since I just had arrived from the US, the microbial community represented by the X dots is a mashup of the US bugs I brought with me and the impact of the food I ate before boarding the plane, the funky in flight food and the food and microbes I acquired while on the ground in Arusha, eating and moving about this new environment. Either way, over those first three days my gut microbial community remained more or less stable (dots are close together suggesting no major shift in the composition of my gut microbiota).

The circle dot represents my first day in the field with the Hadza (for this field session). At this point, I dropped the salads and booze and moved onto a Hadza diet. Since it was late January, we were in the wet season and wild honey and berries were plentiful. I also ate lots of tubers. During this particular field session the Hadza camps we were working in had very little meat, save the occasional bird. In short, they were basically vegetarians. (As a side note, it's important to remember that depending on what time of year a particular anthropologist or ethnographer visits a group around the world (now or in the past), seasonality will have a significant impact on the observed foods being eaten at that point in time

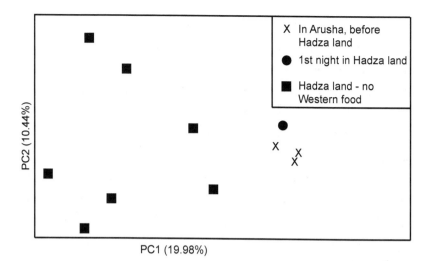

The authors gut microbes - each X, circle and square dot respresents a different day. The closer the dots are together the more similar the gut microbes are together on any particular day.

(and this is more pronounced in lower latitudes). That said, someone visiting the Hadza say 70 years ago (during the same time I was during this field session), would note that their diet was 95% plants. On the flipside, visit the Hadza during November and you would see lots of meat and a different picture of the plant to animal ratio would emerge. I'm just saying).

As the circle dot suggests, my gut microbial community looks pretty much like my US-Arusha gut, but that was about to change. With each passing day in Hadzaland, my microbial community started to shift or more specifically, *reorganize*. With each passing day of eating my new hunter-gatherer vegetarian diet, drinking some pretty suspect water (with the occasional baboon turd floating in it) and cohabitating/mingling with the Hadza on a daily basis (covered in Hadza Land soil), I started to even look less western.

What's important to note here is that my gut microbes didn't start to reorganize during the first few days into a nice little cluster, as we see with my Arusha samples. Instead, I'm all over the place from day to day as my gut lapped up and sampled what was no doubt a mob of new microbes, some sticking around, some not. Since the time points only cover a week or so, it's not known if 1. I would ever settle down (microbially speaking) or 2. how long that would take. I have no doubt, however, that it would settle down, but I'm not sure if I would ever fall into a Hadza cluster, which at this point is still a long way from my moving dots. In addition to my chaotic gut flora during that week, something else and unexpected was happening.

On the opposite page is another plot showing how the diversity of my gut microbiota was shifting as well. The dots are organized left to right and represent the day they were taken. Here again you see my three red dots representing Arusha, then the green dots representing my first day in Hadza land on a Hadza diet. While in Arusha and my first day in Hadza land, the diversity of bacteria in my gut was more or less the same., but then it began to decrease. Around days four and five on the Hadza diet it bottomed out before starting to track slowly upwards. This was totally unexpected.

I originally thought that being in this new, microbially-rich environment, I would quickly acquire a greater diversity of gut bacteria. It's also important to note that I did not participate in the butchering of any animals during this period (as none were killed), but I have no idea if the messiness of butchering would have contributed to my overall gut microbe diversity. In general it seems the diversity of bacteria I brought with me to the field suffered some losses - possibly a combination of flat

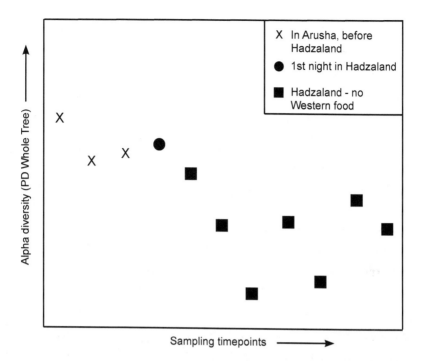

out disappearance or at least lowered to levels not detectable by 16s methods. This could also be a function of diet, i.e. new substrates for the gut microbes to munch on - or being nudged out by new members acquired from this new lifestyle. In either case, the chaotic reorganizing seen in the first graph above suggests that at least in the first few days my losses - for whatever reason - outpaced my acquisition of new members. We know from looking at 100's of Hadza poo samples that the average Hadza harbors nearly *twice the microbial diversity* as my US-Arusha gut. That said, even though my diversity was on the upswing by the end of the week, I had a long way to go before acquiring the diversity we see in the average Hadza.

Interestingly, there were some notable shifts in major groups (Phyla) of microbes. The graph below shows how - at the phylum level - three groups of microbes shifted. As you can see the Firmicutes (red bar) were up and down – nothing too exciting. However, Bacteroidetes and Proteobacteria were definitely on the move.

As for the drop in the phylum Bacteroidetes, the Genus *Bacteroides* seems to account for much of it (see graph). *Bacteroides* are the dominant group of bacteria in the western group. I've suggested that this is *not* a function of our high fat-sugar diet in the west, but rather represents our drop in the quantity and diversity of dietary fiber. If dietary fiber intake goes down, so to does the output of short chain fatty acids from the fermentation of that fiber. This results in a less acidic colonic environment. Since many strains of *Bacteroides* don't like acidity (and grow better in more alkaline environments), then my new diet of copious amounts of fiber from roots and berries would have made my colon more acidic and thus, less inviting for *Bacteroides*. However, I ate virtually no meat during this period so that complicates things a bit - *if* meat/fat/ protein is an important variable. Note that our Hadza data reveal that the Hadza harbor virtually no *Bacteroides*, even during periods of high meat consumption. I did, however, eat mountains of yummy wild honey, larvae and all. On some days I suspect my caloric haul from honey alone ranged from 1,000 to 3,000 calories. Some days I felt like I was going to barf from eating so much of it. Add to these daily handfuls of sweet berries and I was literally bouncing around the landscape.

The significant increase in Proteobacteria can be attributed to a jump in the family of Enterobacteriaceae. This family of gram-negative microbes includes many *harmless symbionts*, but also includes some well-known (and potentially harmful) bugs like e. coli, salmonella, shigella, yersinia and so on. By the last day of sampling, this group of bacteria accounted for an astounding 50% of all the bugs in my gut.

Maybe I should have cut back on the baobab shit water, but as yet I'm not sure of the source. At this point we aren't sure if the increase in my Proteobacteria is harmful or helpful, so stay tuned.

Another interesting shift was also noted in the relative abundance of the genus Akkermansia. Akker has been getting a lot of ink lately in peer-review journals as it's been shown to negatively correlate with obesity[59] (i.e. more Akker is a good thing), and other measures of metabolic health. As a mucin-degrader, Akker helps turn over the mucus layer lining your large bowel and as such, clings closely with your mucus barrier. My Akker levels went from low to none to being a dominant player (though fluctuating).

My shifting levels of Akker are interesting when you consider that the gut bacteria of fasting/hibernating animals like squirrels and periodic-eating pythons[60] is dominated by Akker, or at least Akker increases during periods of reduced nutrient availability. One of the things you quickly notice when on a Hadza diet is that you're hungry. You're not starving or in want of food all the time, but you always feel a little hungry. Interestingly, the Hadza don't jump up in the morning and start eating - remember they don't have refrigeration and limited to zero storage. Unlike us westerners who start eating literally the minute we get up and graze nearly continuously on something throughout the day. The Hadza don't.

I'm going to go out on a limb here and suggest that the Hadza (and presumably our ancestors) were periodically fasters. No news here and I don't mean starving (like argued in the Thrifty Genome Hypothesis). I also don't mean going all day without food as there's plenty of food in Hadza land. Plenty. But rather they don't immediately solve hunger pangs by opening a bag of chips as it takes *just a little bit of effort* to get some food and sometimes you delay your desire to eat because of it. This 'little bit of extra time between mouthfuls' is what I mean by 'intermittent fasting' in the case of the Hadza and what I experienced when I was following the diet. Note that I don't think my Akker levels had anything to do with caloric intake as I was awash in sugary calories thanks to berries and wild honey (and fat from the larvae). This is odd as Akker seems to be associated with how much is coming down the pipe everyday i.e. less substrates in the colon equals greater levels and a relative abundance, of Akker.

So unless my increased levels of Akker are being triggered by something from my new diet and/or somehow I was acquiring them from the environment, then I suspect my (presumably beneficial) increase in Akker had to do with my new foraging lifestyle. Makes you wonder if there might be something to the idea of intermittent fasting, but maybe more correctly thought about from a foraging perspective and not the 'starve yourself for a day' that many put forward in a dizzying number of diet books. It's also interesting to consider that my new high fiber diet, which was minimally processed, may have mechanically scrubbed more Akker from my intestinal wall than my previous diet. This scouring effect would have resulted in more Akker in my stool and thus, more overall abundance. Just a thought and one worth testing at some point.

Paleo vs Vegetarian - who eats more fiber?

I OFTEN HEAR PALEO AND PRIMAL EATERS SAY that their shopping carts almost always look like that of 'a vegetarian grazing through the same supermarket' when it comes to the non-grain veggies it contains. This comment (in my experience) often follows when addressing critics who say that a Paleo/Primal diet focused on fat and protein from animal products means that whole, non-grain plants (and their health-giving fiber) will be significantly reduced. Ancestral eaters time and again respond with *'That is nonsense'* and that such a diet always includes a significant amount of fiber, often *exceeding* that of the average citizen or veggie and grain-focused eater. While I'm generalizing a little here in regards to the ancestral community, let's explore this notion with data from the American Gut project.

The American Gut Project is the largest, open source and crowd-funded microbiome project in the world. I cofounded the project back in 2012 with Rob Knight, who is the scientific leader of the project and now based at University of California-San Diego. The project allows members of the general public an opportunity to peek inside their gut and see who's in there, so long as they donate to the larger citizen science project. As part of American Gut, we suggest that each participant fill out an optional, online questionnaire asking standard things like their age and gender along with questions such as; *do you have any diseases? When was the last time you took antibiotics? Do you brush your teeth? Do you live in a city or a rural setting?* And so on. In addition, we ask them to keep track of the foods they eat for a week by recording the information using an online website that keeps track of calories etc.

Because samples and the data from the questionnaire are self-collected and reported, the American Gut Project is a cross-sectional, observational study. In other words, it's not ideal and it's full of biases (and the researchers running and collaborating on the study are fully aware of this). However, the large number of participants - at the moment >15,000 swabs have been sent out - and the kind of broad questions we are asking of the data, make it an excellent study for accessing the gut microbe variability across the planet for a range of diet and other lifestyle factors. More importantly, the project will help inform future, more detailed studies. Long live citizen science!

Of the 15,000 or so swabs mailed out, not all have been mailed back to the lab, even less have been sequenced and even a smaller amount of those have had the data uploaded. As of this writing, ~4,500 samples have been sequenced with the results uploaded[61]. All publicly available data sets have been de-identified, that is to say 'scrubbed' of any personal information that might link a particular set of results to a particular individual.

As part of the questionnaire we asked people if they were omnivores, vegetarians, vegans and so on. Of the ~4,500 participants with sequenced and uploaded data, ~3,300 of them filled out the questionnaire with enough detail to assess their daily fiber intake based on their food intake for a week. However, from this data we can't tell if a person who has described themselves as an omnivore follows a paleo or primal strategy for eating. For this, I had to try and tease out data from the comments column associated with the dietary info.

Identifying the vegetarians & vegans was easy - they said so. This resulted in 77 vegans and 116 straight up vegetarians. We also had 206 omnivores who don't eat red meat, technically referred to as pescetarian. The truly paleo/primal folks I queried who self-identified as paleo or commented with something like, *'I follow a paleo diet'* or *'I'm primal'* etc. resulted in 73 paleo eaters. For the ones that did not clearly state they followed a paleo/ primal diet but said things like *'I don't eat grains'* or *'I try and follow paleo most of the time,'* I lumped them into a group called 'paleo-like' (n=137). While this is not a perfect way to go about great science, it does separate the non-grain eaters from the vegan & vegetarian folks, (at least for the folks who provided enough info). The distinction of grain eaters vs. non-grain eaters is useful as whole grains contain dietary fiber, (presuming whole grains are what's consumed by our grain eaters (at least some of the time). Below is a box-and-whisker plot of the results.

The median daily fiber intake for our various groups is as follows:

Paleo-Like:	19g/day
Omnivore:	19g/day
Paleo:	25.1g/day

Omnivore, but no red meat: 27.8g/day

Vegetarian: 32.8g/day

Vegan: 43g/day

As you can see - considering our 'not-so-great but interesting cross-sectional observational data' - vegetarians consume more dietary fiber than our paleo folks and vegans beat them all. Our paleo-Like folks didn't do much better than our run-of-the-mill omnivores, who came in at an embarrassing 19 g/day. This is in line with countless studies published over the years about dietary habits of Americans (which suggests that our data is tracking well and thus useful to consider in the *Who eats more fiber?'* theme of this essay).

So on the often-vigorous defense by some in the paleo community that they consume adequate amounts of dietary fiber I call bullshit, at least for this little self-collected data set. I'm not saying that a paleo or paleo-like diet isn't healthy or has been shown in numerous studies to be metabolically beneficial, I'm just saying the paleo folks in this data set consume an embarrassing low amount of dietary fiber by USDA and evolutionary standards. According to the USDA's Dietary Guidelines for Americans[62], adults should be getting 14g/day for every 1,000 calories consumed. If you are on a 2,000-calorie diet, this translates into 28g/day so this means 28-38g/day more or less and depending on your gender. Seems that only our navel-gazing, tofu-slurping vegans surpass government recommendations with their crunchy cuisine. So how does this stack up against our evolutionary past?

I'm often asked what the most striking thing I've experienced or learned while working among the Hadza hunter-gatherers of Tanzania. Aside from their breathtaking contact[63] with the microbial world around them, I would have

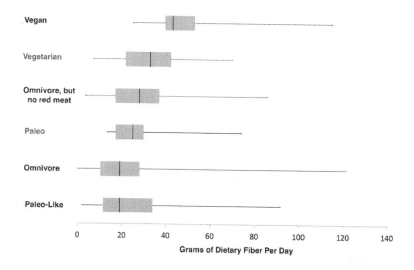

to say their near-constant daily nibbling of dietary fiber was the real eye-opener. Given that the Hadza live in a place in East Africa that presumably gave rise to our genus *Homo* and that they literally hunted and gathered many of the same foods that humans in this region have for millions of years (and are literally covered in the same dirt), their fiber consumption and its impact on their gut microbes has implications for us so-called modern humans in the western world. So given the huge impact dietary fiber has on modulating our intestinal microbes - see Justin and Erica Sonnenburg's new book *The Good Gut* for an exhaustive and well-researched review of the literature on this - the fiber habits of the Hadza are relevant.

As always, I take great pains NOT to get mired into the heated discussions about *'humans evolved and do great on many types of diets'* and *'there is no one Paleo or ancestral diet'* and *'humans haven't stopped evolving and adapting.'* I know this and I get it, but when we are talking about our immune system and the daily tango it plays out with our resident microbes (friend and foe), we can safely assume that a great many of the genes that we carry today - both human *and* microbial genes - were selected in area of the world where we spent most of our time evolving, not only as the genus *Homo* but as members of the larger, ancient primate community. That would be Africa and for the better part of the last few million years, East Africa would be most specifically of interest.

That said, the fiber intake of the Hadza is useful to consider, especially in our work on their gut flora. The published data on Hadza fiber intake is scant and inconsistent[64]. The Hadza consume foods in and outside the camp (often on the go), making it difficult to measure a handful of berries here and a piece of fibrous tuber there, yet as any researcher who has spent time with the Hadza will tell you, fiber intake is 1. high compared to western populations and 2. variable day-to-day and season-to-season[65].

Early researchers and travelers working or visiting Hadza Land commented on the large, distended bellies of many of the Hadza children, often interpreting this as malnutrition. This couldn't be further from the truth. It's a simple function of fermentation of the dietary fiber deep in the bowels of the children. Yes, they eat lots of fiber (but not from 'leafy greens' *per se*). As we've started to quantify the fiber intake among the Hadza, I've been amazed at the amount of fiber the children consume, (and we are still accumulating data). The primary weaning food for Hadza kiddos is the baobab fruit, but maize meal as a weaning food is creeping into more and more families. Mixed with water - and wild honey if available - the concoction of ground baobab flour (highly fibrous, chalky innards with a fat-rich nut inside) from the fruit is consumed daily - yes, daily.

Hardly a day goes by when Hadza women aren't found

digging up fibrous roots or sucking on the chalky and fibrous innards of the baobab and if it's the right time of year, seasonal and fiber-rich berries are consumed in large quantities. As the men walk to and from hunting stands or practice 'encounter hunting' where they walk around for tens of kilometers in a day, they do so while picking small handfuls of various fibrous berries and sucking on fibrous baobab fruit, often just lying on the ground under an endless sea of baobab trees.

As we started quantifying the fiber intake among the Hadza, some surprising and striking patterns began emerging. On any given day, a 4-48 month old kiddo might consume between 30-150g/day of dietary fiber (sometimes more!) and out pops the distended belly (especially among the youngest in the camp). This is directly related to microbial actions deep in their bowels where the microbes go about breaking down the fiber whilst releasing short chain fatty acids, various gases and other byproducts in the process. All of these actions promote the direct growth of some microbes (and the growth of others) through cross-feeding. Again, fiber intake is highly variable.

The adult daily average of fiber intake also varies greatly, but it is high. As children become older and more foods are introduced into their diet (and the young boys start hunting), the ratio of fiber intake to calories consumed seems to drop yet it still sits well above the 14g per 1,000 calories recommended by the USDA. This brings up another interesting question: *why don't USDA dietary guidelines include recommendations for Americans under two years of age?*

I've asked around about this and can't seem to get a clear answer. As best I can tell, it seems to be rooted in some notion that kids under the age of 2 are still consuming some (or a large part) of their daily calories from breast milk, but I could be wrong. As breastfeeding rates have plummeted[66] in the US and elsewhere, this notion seems to be a little outdated.

Even more striking about the Hadza is the nearly constant nibbling of fibrous sources even in the presence of large quantities of other resources like meat and honey - a personal observation. This has huge implications for modern health and well being, specifically with regards to the design of diets in microbial studies. Time and time again, microbial studies finger meaty and sugary diets as having deleterious effects on resident microbial communities in the human gut and therefore the overall health of the host.

Interestingly, these studies will often challenge a group of people or mice with a high fat diet, (not unlike some Hadza gorging on a zebra kill eating the fatty brain and various other organs and marrow), but will not include any fiber - or if they do it's in tiny amounts. While the studies may be mimicking what might be considered 'real world conditions' i.e. the American diet, it ignores our evolutionary past and role of fiber in mitigating/blunting[67] some of the deleterious impact of the fat-fed microbes. Said differently, it would be great to see some studies that challenged mouse and man to high fat diets, but in a mixed meal with evolutionary amounts of fiber. I suspect the outcome would be very different, as would be the headlines of your local paper.

As a side note, the most abundant genera or group of bacteria in the American Gut Project is *Bacteroides* of the phylum Bacteroidetes. In countless studies that see similar findings, it's suggested to be a result of our high fat and sugar American/western diet. Interestingly, *Bacteroides* are a minor group of bacteria in the gut of the Hadza, even during periods of high fat consumption during the dry season when animals are easier to kill, as well as during periods when they eat tons of sugar (as honey and sugary berries are more abundant in wetter periods). Since some species of *Bacteroides* are pH sensitive, i.e. the more acidity the *less Bacteroides* you might see, then we might expect to see less in the Hadza as the higher fiber diet means more fermentation which translates into more things like short chain fatty acids and greater acidity. And that's exactly what we do see but at this point, we don't know the true reason for the lower abundance of *Bacteroides* in the Hadza gut.

Another side note: it's hard to wrap my head around the idea that sugar intake has such a huge impact on the distal gut microflora, as sugar and its relatives are actually absorbed in the upper GI tract - *before* it reaches the colon and *could* have an impact on the distal gut microbes. This isn't well understood and would be interesting if it were explored in a little more detail. Maybe it's a downstream effect i.e. it shifts the communities in the upper GI, which in turn have a downstream impact on the more distal communities of microbes in the colon. Maybe it's the absence of the low intake of fiber because the sugary things make up the larger portion of the diet, that is the bigger issue/problem. I.e. it's not what we are eating but what we are *not* eating, which is fiber.

Paleo brothers and sisters you need to get your shit together (pun intended) and start trying to eat more fiber if you want to truly eat a more microbially relevant ancestral diet[68]. That goes for all of us. If you don't or can't eat more fiber than even the most ardent among the ancestral movement should be labeled paleo-like or paleo-*lite*.

In closing, us so-called modern humans probably have the most alkaline guts in human history, simply because we don't eat enough fiber - not even close. I'm gonna go out on a limb here and suggest that the big bellies of these Hadza kids are trying to tell us something about the importance of an acidic colonic environment early in our development - specifically in this 4-6 month window when they (and presumably all of us) started receiving our first non-breastmilk foods. This, coupled with their microbially-rich environment, in contrast to the hyper-sterile environment our kids live in today, may hold the clues to the rise of some of the terrible diseases our children are afflicted with so early in life. If this die is cast early in our immune system development then it has implications for our health as adults as well.

If I had to pick one thing among the myriad of dietary decisions we are faced with on a daily or weekly basis, making our colonic environment *more acidic* would be at the top of the list. By doing so, our more acidic colons will mean better barrier function (less leaky gut) and a more hostile environment for potentially pathogenic bacteria, plus a greater diversity of microbes. Smile. Your next meal is fast approaching.

Please note I do not have an agenda with this article. As anyone who reads my writing knows, I'm a big fan of all things paleo, as well as a big-time eater of all things flesh.

Swapping microbes
with your dog

WE HUG THEM, KISS THEM, SLEEP WITH THEM
and share our food with them. They are, of course, the family
dog. In return, they share with us some of the microbes they
pick up as they saunter about the neighborhood and places
beyond. A study conducted by researchers at the University
of Colorado-Boulder reveals those families who own dogs
harbor a more diverse and different set of skin bacteria than
non-dog owning families. More importantly, the microbial
exchange that takes place during the slobbering and paw-
petting ritual of canine companionship reminds us of
some time-honored interactions with the ancient and very
microbial landscape that our western world and culture has
walled off, and possibly not in a good way.

Following the observation that the gut microbiota
of monozygotic twins (identical twins) are not any more
similar than dizygotic twins (fraternal), (suggesting that

more than genetics determines the selection and source of the microbes on and in your body), the Colorado researchers wanted to explore how co-habiting with other family members and dogs shaped host microbiota. In other words; *how does environmental exposure to other people (related and unrelated) and other species (dogs) shape your microbial ecology?*

The researchers collected stool, oral and skin (forehead, right and left palm) samples (swabs) of the humans and the same for the dogs, except all four paws of the dogs were sampled. In all, they studied 159 individuals[69] and 36 dogs.

Group 1: 17 families with children aged 6 to 18 yrs of age
Group 2: 17 families with one or more dogs, but no children
Group 3: 8 families with children and dogs
Group 4: 18 families with no kids or dogs

Not surprisingly, the researchers found that family units share similar microbial communities at all sites sampled (stool, skin & oral). The skin was the most similar between family members, as family members often interact with the same objects and surfaces in a home. They also found that parents share similar oral (tongue) and gut communities with children aged 3-18 years in the home, but less so with children <3 years of age - a pattern seen in studies of other populations[70] throughout the world, which reveals the dynamic and still maturing nature of the infant oral and gut ecosystem.

They also found that cohabiting partners shared more microbes with one another than say the neighbors next door. They also found that on average, about 11% of the bacteria on someone's hands (palms) was likely to be from oral sources, while less than 2% was from fecal sources. In both cases, it demonstrates the movement of bacteria between various body sites, which are also ultimately shared with your partner.

They also found that the sharing of microbes between partners is also mimicked with dogs. They found that dog owners share more skin bacteria (skin to paw) with their own dogs than say with the neighbor's dogs but the similarities between human and dog were less pronounced in infants and seniors, possibly suggesting 'behavioral differences between age groups.'

In an interesting twist, they found that couples who own a dog share more skin (palm and forehead) microbes between each other than couples who do not have a dog. Conversely, people who live together but do not have a dog, look less similar to one another. In other words, the dog is the great equalizer and source of rare and novel microbes that are passed on to their human companions. Side note: adult females have a greater diversity of bacteria on their hands than do males. Second side note: cats in the house (cats weren't sampled) had no effect on the diversity of skin bacteria among adults. In addition to

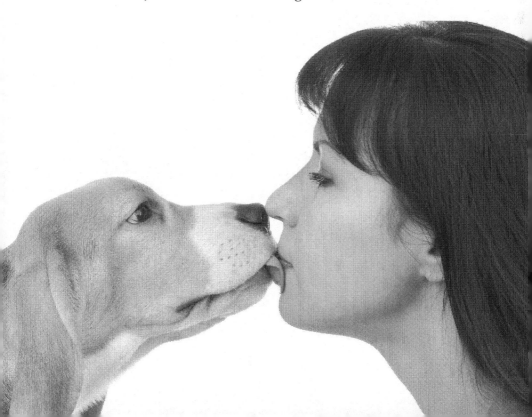

this, dog-owning adults seem to share more skin microbes with their dogs than they do with their children.   Unlike skin microbial communities, dog ownership had no effect on oral and gut communities in humans. Increasing family size had a significant effect on shared skin microbial communities, i.e. the bigger the family the more homogenizing of the skin communities amongst everyone in the house.

In closing, the researchers note that much of the similarity between the skin microbiota of humans and their dogs can be explained by the oral-skin transfer, aka licking. In addition, a number of the taxa identified on the paws and forehead of the dogs are commonly associated with soil and water, which the dogs in turn track into the house and onto their owners. The paw and forehead of dogs also showed a greater diversity and evenness of bacteria, consistent with their frequent exposure to a great number of microbial sources.

All in all, the study reveals that our pets harbor a diverse microbial community that ultimately can influence our own microbial community structure and thus, our health. The same goes for the people we cohabitate with as well, via their collective and shared exposure outside the home. It's not much of a stretch to imagine that our overall broad exposure to the larger microbial world has decreased in our modern world. While some of this may be a good thing, we may be depriving our host-associated microbial ecosystems from some health-giving diversity that was once the norm throughout human evolution. In all things ecological, diversity is a good thing. If you want to channel your ancestors for some wisdom, you might start by hugging an animal (or two) and getting outside a little more often.

Slumdog Microbiome
are More Diverse

I WAS RECENTLY INVITED TO PUT TOGETHER a series of slides for a national supermarket chain on things their customers could do to improve the health of their gut microbiome. Once I got past the obvious first few slides that recommend they might spend a little less time in national supermarket chains and get someone smarter than me to do the webinar, I listed what I think is the most important. The most counterintuitive recommendation that was still in keeping with my only half-kidding slides up until this point? Move to a slum in Bangladesh.

As researchers plumb the gut of an increasing number of non-western or so-called 'developing regions and nations' throughout the world, an interesting pattern is emerging. Not unexpectedly, different populations harbor different combinations of bacteria on their skin[71] and in their bowels[72].

They also have a greater overall diversity of bacteria. When it comes to our inner ecosystem, our kick-it-and-see western diet and lifestyle experiment may not only be removing some important members altogether, (think widespread use of antibiotics, for example), but actually reducing our gut microbiome's ability to defend itself (and us) against opportunistic pathogens (some domestic, some foreign) and reducing its overall metabolic output. (More on this in a minute).

A recent study[73] comparing healthy children from the slums of Bangladesh with children in the U.S. is adding to a growing body of literature suggesting that we may be getting a little too clean for our own good. In this study they collected stool samples from six healthy Bangladeshi children (ages 8-13), four healthy U.S. children (ages 10-14) and four Bangladeshi adults (ages 18-41). rDNA pyrosequencing was performed on all the samples, which provided a detail of the microbes present and their abundance in each of the samples. In addition, they also wanted to see how the gut microbiome changed overtime, so they collected monthly samples for five months from four of the six Bangladeshi children and for six months from all four of the U.S. children.

Overall, the Bangladeshi children harbored a greater diversity of gut bacteria than did their U.S. counterparts. This finding is similar to that reported between children living in a rural African village in Burkina Faso[74], when compared to children in Italy. This same diversity disparity is also noted between Venezuelan Amazonas and rural Malawians when compared[75] to U.S. populations - of all ages. In addition, while the kiddos in the U.S. carried some bacterial genera (n=3) not seen in the Bangladeshi kids, the Bangladeshi kids carried many more (n=13) *not found* in the U.S. children.

The diet between the two populations could not be

more different. In the U.S., the children consume much more protein and fat from animal resources, while the kids in Bangladesh rarely eat meat, but have a diet based on lentils, bread and rice. The researchers also speculate that the U.S. kids have a more diverse diet, although detailed dietary information was not collected as part of the study.

What was potentially more interesting was how the gut microbiome changed over time. In short, the Bangladeshi kids showed greater diversity from month to month (from the baseline of the original sample) than the U.S. kids - i.e. they were more stable-like.

The take home from this small but interesting study is potentially profound. While the researchers are quick to point out that the 'causal relationships underlying the composition changes' are difficult to pinpoint - genetics, diet and lifestyle all play a likely role. From the perspective of an ecologist and more specifically, a microbial ecologists' - diversity is something you really want in an ecosystem. Greater diversity is associated with resilience, or the microbiomes ability to deal with such things as opportunistic pathogens or perturbations from one's diet. A less biodiverse gut microbiome may handle your five-donut binge at the office or your bottle and half of red wine one night (instead of your usual two glasses), *very differently*. Dietary pulses (or longer term shifts in diet such as antibiotic use) are perturbations that can shift the composition of your gut microbiome and reduce diversity, as some species become more dominant under the perturbation.

The greater month-to-month variability in bacteria in the Bangladeshi kids is not likely attributable to a lack of antibiotics or wide shifts in diet. It is likely the continuous and intensive exposure to a diversity of microbes in their environment (due to varying unhygienic conditions found in the slum), that is driving the diversity. The potential greater exposure to large swaths of diverse people and animals contribute as well - something that has been lost in more western societies.

Infectious disease and associated gastroenteritis can be rampant (and deadly) in developing countries, revealing that the factors that shape microbial diversity and one's susceptibility to disease are complex. But the emerging themes of diversity and our ancestral lifestyle of constant exposure to the natural world and its myriad of wonderful (but sometimes harmful) microbes will likely dominate our discussions of health and wellbeing in the decades to come - at least I hope they will.

Palm Oil: maybe not such a good diea after all

THERE ARE TWO THINGS THAT YOU CAN BE certain of when it comes to palm oil: 1. business is booming and 2. orangutans hate palm oil. If they could speak to us, I'm pretty confident that's what they would say. We can now add another certainty to that: palm oil causes low-grade inflammation that is linked to insulin resistance, obesity and other metabolic diseases that are partially mediated by our resident gut microbes.

Palm oil is touted as a panacea for everything ranging from a route out of poverty for small-scale farmers, a sustainable biofuel and for its powerful nutritional virtues as well. However, palm oil plantations are linked to unsustainable deforestation[76] throughout the world and this (aside from the obvious biosphere issues), is reducing the livable habitat for orangutans to the point that some are calling it genocide.

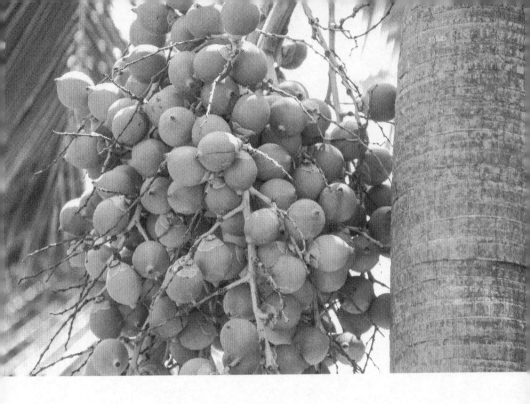

Consumer demand (or maybe that should be 'manufacturer demand'), for palm oil has resulted in palm oil appearing in one of every two packaged products in the supermarket. You can find it in baked goods, cereals, crisps, sweets, margarine, popular soaps and cosmetics - to name a few. Often listed under a dizzying number of names like 'palmate' and 'sodium lauryl sulphate', it's not always easy to spot. Red palm oil has become very popular among the more affluent, both for its taste, cool red color and superior antioxidant load. The red palm oil is derived from the fleshy part of the fruit - hence its red color - while the clear stuff comes from the whitish kernel in the center. You can also refine red palm oil down to a 'clear version' (but in the process, you lose some of its goodness).

I have discussed elsewhere the potential impact of a high-fat diet and changes in your gut microbial ecosystem that can (and does) lead to low-grade inflammation that furthers leads to insulin resistance, obesity and other issues. In short, high-fat intake shifts the gut microbiota and increases the translocation of lipopolysaccharides (LPS) or endotoxins from your gut into your blood, which then triggers inflammation - and then the cascade of problems start.

These 'high-fat-increases-endotoxin-load-in-serum' studies used varying amounts and types of fat, with no particular emphasis on the type of fat being used. These researchers also, due to the nature of the research and the questions being asked, used what some might consider unrealistic levels of fat in the mouse or human diet being tested - levels you would not see in any free-living human population. This research reality is simply a function of the researchers exploring cause and effect and in order to do so, the need to 'dial it up' a bit to get any meaningful shifts in the data. In either case, the outcomes are still informative.

Researchers in France decided to address both of these issues in a recent study[77] among mice fed proportional and realistic levels of fat and tested oils with differing fatty acid composition (albeit in mice). The fats/oils tested included milk fat, palm oil, rapeseed (canola) oil and sunflower oil.

Regardless of which fat the mice received, fat content as a percentage of diet was maintained at 22.4% (or 38% of the *energy* of the diet). Mice were randomly divided into five groups (8 mice per group) and fed one of the five diets (one was a control i.e. normal mice chow food *not* spiked with fat). Fast forwarding a bit, the researchers found that depending on which oil the mice received, it could change the levels of endotoxins in their serum (impaired gut) and increase markers of inflammation - not so good.

Turns out that compared to a high-fat diet formulated

with either milk fat, rapeseed oil or sunflower oil, the one that included palm oil resulted in higher inflammation in both plasma and adipose tissue, as measured by a number of markers. Interestingly, rapeseed oil resulted in much lower inflammation. (Would encourage folks that are interested in the subject to read the detailed and related studies themselves).

In this study, researchers used refined, non-hydrogenated palm oil (and not oil from the kernel). That is, red palm oil without the 'red'. If you are concerned about low-grade inflammation then you might want to think twice about forking out the extra money for the fancy palm oil. You might want to check the ingredient labels a little more closely as well.

Maybe it doesn't matter at all. Maybe the differences between the inflammation triggered by one fatty acid over the other is insignificant. Maybe they should have used more mice or heated the oil. Maybe mouse studies don't matter. Maybe more studies are needed.

In either case, thinking twice about palm oil might please the orangutans.

American (Gut) Gothic: 5 things you can do for a healthier microbiome in 2015

IN THE SUMMER OF 2008, A 26-YEAR-OLD MAN from Shanxi Province walked into a lab at Shanghai Jiao Tong University. 23 weeks later he walked out 113 pounds lighter. He had not participated in a clinical trial of some new secret weight loss pill, nor had he signed up for a punishing Biggest Loser-style exercise program, nor was he fussed over by behavioral scientists who made his plates and drinking cups smaller with each passing week. The researchers (who were microbiologists) had simply put the man's gut microbes on a diet.

One of the huge mysteries in studies of diet and exercise is the remarkable difference in outcomes between individuals who get the very same treatment. Inevitably, some people in a study show little improvement despite weeks (or even months) of following what might seem like draconian changes in their normal diet and lifestyle. Other people apparently drop weight just by getting out of bed in the morning and also end up improving their circulating triglycerides, total cholesterol and biomarkers of inflammation with apparent ease. We all know someone like this from our daily lives.

So why are there such extreme differences between these people? Is our DNA to blame?

Our human genes *may* be involved in some cases but we generally share more than 99% genetic similarity with other people. More interestingly, the huge differences in people's weight gain/loss may be driven more by the different bacteria in their intestines, which can be more than 90% different between one person and the next.

In addition to the familiar human genome we inherit from our moms and dads, each of us also have hundreds of trillions of microbial symbionts, each with their own genomes. Research programs such as the Human Microbiome Project[78] have revolutionized our understanding of our microbial bodies, which outnumber our human cells ten to one and account for more than 2 pounds of our body weight. We know microbes can change profoundly in each of us throughout our lives and that we can also change them through diet, medications, hygiene etc. We also now know that how we enter this world[79] - C-section versus vaginal birth - can impact a human being's initial 'seeding' of microbes, which further change during breast (or formula) feeding. We know too that what you eat later in life affects your gut microbes and even how healthy you are as a senior citizen[80]. We know that people in more traditional societies[81] have different microbes than those in more Westernized populations and that diet can play a significant role in these differences. You can also change the health prospects of a mouse overnight by changing its diet and thus, its microbes.

Advances in bioinformatics (a fancy word for 'data analysis'), and refinements of DNA techniques (not to mention a significant increase in computing power), is changing everything. The evidence that life events and diet can shape our gut microbes is increasing, but which direction should we be nudging them? What exactly *is* a healthy and optimal mix of gut microbes? The honest answer is nobody knows (yet), but projects are underway (e.g., American Gut) that you can participate in, to help us to better understand the role bacteria play in our health and well-being.

In the meantime, as you contemplate your New Year resolutions to join the gym, lose weight, improve your diet or to purchase the latest gizmo to track your every move, you might want to consider whether your microbes will support your decision. After all, they're the one's actually *in control,* so take that you anthropocentric ape!

Below are five suggestions on how you might improve the health of your gut microbes (and some other microbes in your life).

No. 5. Antibiotics. It's a familiar story by now: over zealous use of antibiotics are driving antibiotic resistance among microbes at an alarming rate, but it gets worse. The average child in the developed world will likely receive 10-20 courses of antibiotics before his or her 18th birthday. This, coupled with the low therapeutic doses[82] in animal feed (and therefore, our feed), may be shifting our gut microbes into an unhealthy state and possibly contributing to the metabolic disease of obesity. It's also well documented that following a course of broad-spectrum antibiotics, it could take weeks, months or even years for your gut microbial community to bounce back - if at all. During this period of imbalance, opportunistic pathogens can set up shop, or worse. While antibiotics are clearly needed in some (probably most) scenarios, ask more questions before downing them without at least some consideration.

No. 4. Open a window. For 99.99% of human history, the outside was always part of the inside, and at no moment during our day were we ever really separated from nature. Today, a National Activity Survey[83] found that between enclosed buildings and vehicles, modern humans spend a whopping 90% of their lives indoors. Though keeping the outside out does have its advantages such as protection from the elements and decreasing your chances of being eaten by a zombie, it has also changed the microbiome of our home. Studies[84] show that maybe opening a window and increasing the natural airflow will improve the diversity and health of the microbes in your home, which in turn benefit its inhabitants. In the not-so-distant future, building codes will likely reflect the biological benefits of rewilding our living and workspaces. Never hurts to get a head start.

No. 3. Adopt an ecological perspective. Familiarize yourself with the writings of Aldo Leopold, John Muir and other important and interesting naturalists and ecologists, past and present. The human-microbial superorganism is a vast ecological system, subject to the same rules of resistance, resilience and balance as any ecosystem on the planet. The sooner you learn to tend your microbial garden[85], the sooner you will understand how human ecology and your health is nothing more than understanding our history and place in the larger biosphere[86]. Google the word Anthropocene - you would do well to understand it's meaning and potential impact on your microbes and the world around you.

No. 2. Eat more plants. This is not a hard one and I don't

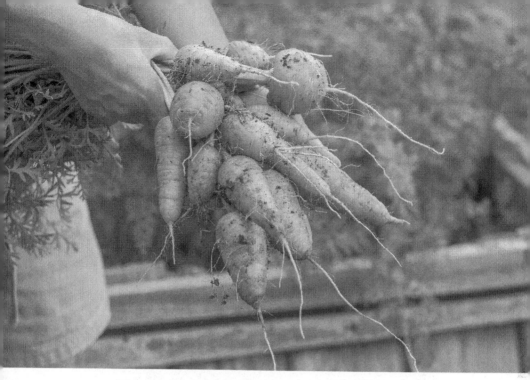

Getting dirty has never been more important.

mean 'give up meat,' but I *do* mean to eat a greater diversity and quantity of whole plants. In my opinion this is the single most important dietary strategy for improving the diversity and health of your gut microbiome. In short, your gut microbes thrive on a diversity of fermentable substrates (aka *dietary fiber*). But not all fiber is made the same (physically or chemically); so consuming a diversity of whole plants will assure a steady flow of substrates for your resident microbes. Also, make sure you eat more of the whole plant and not just the soft and tasty parts. Consume the entire asparagus, not just the tip. Consume the trunk of the broccoli, not just the crown. Consume all of the greens at the top of the leek, not just the bulb. By doing so, you will guarantee that the harder-to-digest portions of the plant will extend the metabolic activity of your microbiome deep into your bowels. Also, track how many species of plants you eat in a week and shoot for 30-40 or more.

No. 1. Get your hands dirty. More to the point; *start a garden or something similar.* Getting your hands dirty and covering more of your body (and food) with mother nature's blanket will help you not only connect with the natural world we have tried so hard to remove ourselves from, but will reacquaint your immune system with the trillions of microorganisms on the plants and in the soil. The loss of this interface with the *terra firma* of our evolutionary past - body to soil, body to nature - is where the wheels really came off the wagon. As people of the world move from poverty to middle class, they also move from the gritty realities of our ancestral life to the promise of modern development with its triple-washed produce and squeaky-clean surroundings. Reconnecting with ecosystems, through gardening or some other 'outside' means will allow you to understand and manage your very own inner-ecosystem. There's really no better way.

NOTES

1   Costello EK, Stagaman K, Dethlefsen L, Bohannan BJM, Relman DA. The application of ecological theory towards an understanding of the human microbiome. *Science (New York, NY)*. 2012;336(6086):1255-1262. doi:10.1126/science.1224203.

2   van Nood, E., et al. (2013). "Duodenal Infusion of Donor Feces for Recurrent Clostridium difficile." *New England Journal of Medicine* **368**(5): 407-415.

3   Prufer, K., et al. (2012). "The bonobo genome compared with the chimpanzee and human genomes." *Nature* **486**(7404): 527-531.

4   Nielsen R, Bustamante C, Clark AG, Glanowski S, Sackton TB, Hubisz MJ, et al. (2005) A Scan for Positively Selected Genes in the Genomes of Humans and Chimpanzees. *PLoS Biol* 3(6): e170.

5   Degnan, P. H., et al. (2012). "Factors associated with the diversification of the gut microbial communities within chimpanzees from Gombe National Park." *Proceedings of the National Academy of Sciences* **109**(32): 13034-13039.

6   Stanford, C. B. (1996). "The Hunting Ecology of Wild Chimpanzees: Implications for the Evolutionary Ecology of Pliocene Hominids." *American Anthropologist* **98**(1): 96-113.

7   Stanford, C. B. (1996). "The Hunting Ecology of Wild

Chimpanzees: Implications for the Evolutionary Ecology of Pliocene Hominids." *American Anthropologist* **98**(1): 96-113.

8   http://ngm.nationalgeographic.com/2008/04/chimps-with-spears/mary-roach-text

9   Barreiro, L. B., et al. (2010). "Functional Comparison of Innate Immune Signaling Pathways in Primates." PLoS Genet **6**(12)

10   Yatsunenko, T., et al. (2012). "Human gut microbiome viewed across age and geography." Nature **486**(7402): 222-227.

11   De Filippo, C., et al. (2010). "Impact of diet in shaping gut microbiota revealed by a comparative study in children from Europe and rural Africa." Proceedings of the National Academy of Sciences **107**(33): 14691-14696.

12   http://phylogenomics.wordpress.com/

13   Koeth, R. A., et al. (2013). "Intestinal microbiota metabolism of L-carnitine, a nutrient in red meat, promotes atherosclerosis." Nat Med **19**(5): 576-585.

14   http://www.howjsay.com/index.php?word=carnitine

15   http://www.ncbi.nlm.nih.gov/pubmed/20071648

16   http://humanfoodproject.com/americangut/

17   Dethlefsen, L. and D. A. Relman (2011). "Incomplete recovery and individualized responses of the human distal gut microbiota to repeated antibiotic perturbation." Proceedings

of the National Academy of Sciences **108**(Supplement 1): 4554-4561.

18   Zimmer, J., et al. (2012). "A vegan or vegetarian diet substantially alters the human colonic faecal microbiota." Eur J Clin Nutr **66**(1): 53-60.

19   Koren, O., et al. (2013). "A Guide to Enterotypes across the Human Body: Meta-Analysis of Microbial Community Structures in Human Microbiome Datasets." PLoS Computational Biology **9**(1): e1002863.

20   The 1,000 steaks a day was calculated by Dr. Chris Masterjohn in a very clever blog post (http://www.westonaprice. org/blogs/cmasterjohn/2013/04/10/does-carnitine-from-red-meat-contribute-to-heart-disease-through-intestinal-bacterial-metabolism-to-tmao/). Highly recommended.

21   Purushe, J., et al. (2010). "Comparative genome analysis of *Prevotella* ruminicola and *Prevotella* bryantii: insights into their environmental niche." Microb Ecol **60**(4): 721-729.

22   Lappi, J., et al. (2013). "Intake of whole-grain and fiber-rich rye bread versus refined wheat bread does not differentiate intestinal microbiota composition in Finnish adults with metabolic syndrome." J Nutr **143**(5): 648-655.

23   Martinez, I., et al. (2013). "Gut microbiome composition is linked to whole grain-induced immunological improvements." ISME J **7**(2): 269-280.

24   Martínez, I., et al. (2010). "Resistant Starches Types

2 and 4 Have Differential Effects on the Composition of the Fecal Microbiota in Human Subjects." PLoS ONE **5**(11): e15046.

25   Wu, G. D., et al. (2011). "Linking long-term dietary patterns with gut microbial enterotypes." Science **334**(6052): 105-108.

26   Beards, E., et al. (2010). "Bacterial, SCFA and gas profiles of a range of food ingredients following in vitro fermentation by human colonic microbiota." Anaerobe **16**(4): 420-425.

Shen, Q., et al. (2012). "High-level dietary fibre up-regulates colonic fermentation and relative abundance of saccharolytic bacteria within the human faecal microbiota in vitro." Eur J Nutr **51**(6): 693-705.

Krajmalnik-Brown, R., et al. (2012). "Effects of gut microbes on nutrient absorption and energy regulation." Nutr Clin Pract **27**(2): 201-214.

Arora, T., et al. (2012). "Differential effects of two fermentable carbohydrates on central appetite regulation and body composition." PLoS ONE **7**(8): e43263.

Jumpertz, R., et al. (2011). "Energy-balance studies reveal associations between gut microbes, caloric load, and nutrient absorption in humans." Am J Clin Nutr **94**(1): 58-65.

Lesmes, U., et al. (2008). "Effects of Resistant Starch Type III Polymorphs on Human Colon Microbiota and Short Chain

Fatty Acids in Human Gut Models." Journal of Agricultural and Food Chemistry 56(13): 5415-5421.

Blaut, M. (2002). "Relationship of prebiotics and food to intestinal microflora." Eur J Nutr 41 Suppl 1: I11-16.

Saulnier, D. M., et al. (2009). "Microbiology of the human intestinal tract and approaches for its dietary modulation." Curr Pharm Des 15(13): 1403-1414.

27   El Kaoutari, A., et al. (2013). "The abundance and variety of carbohydrate-active enzymes in the human gut microbiota." Nat Rev Microbiol 11(7): 497-504.

28   Everard, A., et al. (2013). "Cross-talk between Akkermansia muciniphila and intestinal epithelium controls diet-induced obesity." Proceedings of the National Academy of Sciences of the United States of America 110(22): 9066-9071.

29   Duncan, S. H., et al. (2009). "The role of pH in determining the species composition of the human colonic microbiota." Environ Microbiol 11(8): 2112-2122.

30   Hernandez, E., et al. (2013). "Functional consequences of microbial shifts in the human gastrointestinal tract linked to antibiotic treatment and obesity." Gut Microbes 4(4): 306-315.

31   Duncan, S. H., et al. (2009). "The role of pH in determining the species composition of the human colonic microbiota." Environ Microbiol 11(8): 2112-2122.

32   http://www.ncbi.nlm.nih.gov/pmc/articles/

PMC1828662/pdf/2340-06.pdf

33   Kumari, R., et al. (2013). "Fluctuations in butyrate-producing bacteria in ulcerative colitis patients of North India." World J Gastroenterol **19**(22): 3404-3414.

34   Wu, N., et al. (2013). "Dysbiosis signature of fecal microbiota in colorectal cancer patients." Microb Ecol **66**(2): 462-470.

35   Cani, P. D., et al. (2012). "Involvement of gut microbiota in the development of low-grade inflammation and type 2 diabetes associated with obesity." Gut Microbes **3**(4): 279-288.

36   Cani, P. D. and N. M. Delzenne (2010). "Involvement of the gut microbiota in the development of low grade inflammation associated with obesity: focus on this neglected partner." Acta Gastroenterol Belg **73**(2): 267-269.

37   Ridaura, V. K., et al. (2013). "Gut Microbiota from Twins Discordant for Obesity Modulate Metabolism in Mice." Science **341**(6150).

38   http://www.earthmicrobiome.org/

39   Wu, G. D., et al. (2011). "Linking Long-Term Dietary Patterns with Gut Microbial Enterotypes." Science **334**(6052): 105-108.

40   Lozupone, C. A., et al. (2013). "Alterations in the

gut microbiota associated with HIV-1 infection." Cell Host Microbe **14**(3): 329-339.

41   Scher, J. U., et al. (2013). "Expansion of intestinal *Prevotella* copri correlates with enhanced susceptibility to arthritis." Elife **2**: e01202.

42   Kang, D.-W., et al. (2013). "Reduced Incidence of <italic>Prevotella</italic> and Other Fermenters in Intestinal Microflora of Autistic Children." PLoS ONE **8**(7): e68322.

43   Duncan, S. H., et al. (2009). "The role of pH in determining the species composition of the human colonic microbiota." Environ Microbiol **11**(8): 2112-2122.

44   Lin, A., et al. (2013). "Distinct Distal Gut Microbiome Diversity and Composition in Healthy Children from Bangladesh and the United States." PLoS ONE **8**(1): e53838.

45   Trompette, A., et al. (2014). "Gut microbiota metabolism of dietary fiber influences allergic airway disease and hematopoiesis." Nat Med **20**(2): 159-166.

46   David, L. A., et al. (2014). "Diet rapidly and reproducibly alters the human gut microbiome." Nature **505**(7484): 559-563.

47
http://humanfoodproject.com/wp-content/uploads/2014/01/Science_NewsFocus_Leach.pdf

48
http://humanfoodproject.com/wp-content/

uploads/2013/12/Nature_blurb_hadza.pdf

49   http://health.usnews.com/best-diet

50   Potts, R. (2012). "Environmental and Behavioral Evidence Pertaining to the Evolution of Early Homo." Current Anthropology 53(S6): S299-S317.

51   http://newswatch.nationalgeographic.com/blog/ rising-star-expedition/

52   http://www.yourwildlife.org/2013/12/revealing-the-twenty-most-important-species-living-in-your-body/

53   Wu, G. D., et al. (2011). "Linking long-term dietary patterns with gut microbial enterotypes." Science 334(6052): 105-108.

54   Hayashi, H., et al. (2007). "*Prevotella* copri sp. nov. and *Prevotella* stercorea sp. nov., isolated from human faeces." Int J Syst Evol Microbiol 57(Pt 5): 941-946.

55   Scher, J. U., et al. (2013). "Expansion of intestinal *Prevotella* copri correlates with enhanced susceptibility to arthritis." Elife 2: e01202.

56   Lozupone, C. A., et al. (2014). "HIV-induced alteration in gut microbiota: driving factors, consequences, and effects of antiretroviral therapy." Gut Microbes 5(4): 562-570.

57   Siener, R., et al. (2013). "The role of Oxalobacter formigenes colonization in calcium oxalate stone disease." Kidney Int 83(6): 1144-1149.

58   Blaser, M. J. and S. Falkow (2009). "What are the consequences of the disappearing human microbiota?" Nat Rev Microbiol **7**(12): 887-894.

59   Everard, A., et al. (2013). "Cross-talk between Akkermansia muciniphila and intestinal epithelium controls diet-induced obesity." Proceedings of the National Academy of Sciences of the United States of America **110**(22): 9066-9071.

60   Costello, E. K., et al. (2010). "Postprandial remodeling of the gut microbiota in Burmese pythons." ISME J **4**(11): 1375-1385.

61   https://github.com/biocore/American-Gut/tree/master/data

62   http://www.health.gov/dietaryguidelines/

63   Leach, J. (2013). "Gut microbiota: Please pass the microbes." Nature **504**(7478): 33-33.

64   http://www.bec.ucla.edu/papers/Schoeninger2.pdf

65   Berbesque, J. C., et al. (2011). "Sex differences in Hadza eating frequency by food type." Am J Hum Biol **23**(3): 339-345.

66   Allen, J. A., et al. (2015). "Breastfeeding Supportive Hospital Practices in the US Differ by County Urbanization Level." J Hum Lact **31**(3): 440-443.

67   Cani, P. D., et al. (2012). "Involvement of gut microbiota in the development of low-grade inflammation and type 2 diabetes associated with obesity." <u>Gut Microbes</u> **3**(4): 279-288.

68   https://www.psychologytoday.com/blog/the-good-gut/201507/is-your-microbiome-paleo-diet

69   http://elife.elifesciences.org/content/2/e00458

70   Yatsunenko, T., et al. (2012). "Human gut microbiome viewed across age and geography." <u>Nature</u> **486**(7402): 222-227.

71   Trivedi, B. (2012). "Microbiome: The surface brigade." <u>Nature</u> **492**(7429): S60-S61.

72   Yatsunenko, T., et al. (2012). "Human gut microbiome viewed across age and geography." <u>Nature</u> **486**(7402): 222-227.

73   Lin, A., et al. (2013). "Distinct Distal Gut Microbiome Diversity and Composition in Healthy Children from Bangladesh and the United States." <u>PLoS ONE</u> **8**(1): e53838.

74   De Filippo, C., et al. (2010). "Impact of diet in shaping gut microbiota revealed by a comparative study in children from Europe and rural Africa." <u>Proceedings of the National Academy of Sciences</u> **107**(33): 14691-14696.

75   Yatsunenko, T., et al. (2012). "Human gut microbiome viewed across age and geography." <u>Nature</u> **486**(7402): 222-227.

76   Carlson, K. M., et al. (2012). "Committed carbon emissions, deforestation, and community land conversion from oil palm plantation expansion in West Kalimantan, Indonesia." Proceedings of the National Academy of Sciences **109**(19): 7559-7564.

77   Laugerette, F., et al. (2012). "Oil composition of high-fat diet affects metabolic inflammation differently in connection with endotoxin receptors in mice." Am J Physiol Endocrinol Metab **302**(3): E374-386.

78   http://www.hmpdacc.org/

79   http://humanfoodproject.com/kids-are-mammals-time-we-treated-treating-them-like-it/

80   http://humanfoodproject.com/what-can-a-100-year-old-irish-grandmother-teach-us-about-school-lunches/

81   http://www.nature.com/nature/journal/v486/n7402/abs/nature11053.html

82   Cho, I., et al. (2012). "Antibiotics in early life alter the murine colonic microbiome and adiposity." Nature **488**(7413): 621-626.

83   Klepeis, N. E., et al. (2001). "The National Human Activity Pattern Survey (NHAPS): a resource for assessing exposure to environmental pollutants." J Expo Anal Environ Epidemiol **11**(3): 231-252.

84   Kembel, S. W., et al. (2012). "Architectural design influences the diversity and structure of the built environment microbiome." <u>ISME J</u> **6**(8): 1469-1479.

85   http://www.nytimes.com/2012/06/19/science/ studies-of-human-microbiome-yield-new-insights. html?pagewanted=all

86   http://humanfoodproject.com/are-you-there-al-gore-its-me-microbiome/

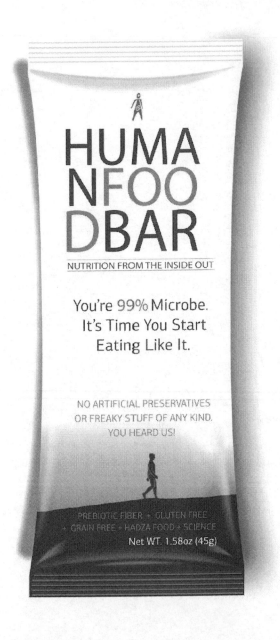

www.humanfoodbar.com

A percentage of proceeds go to support our
work in Africa and Mongolia.

Made in the USA
Lexington, KY
10 November 2017